ADDITIVE MIGRATION
FROM PLASTICS INTO FOOD

Other Titles of Interest

CROMPTON, T. R.
Analysis of Organoaluminium and Organozinc Compounds

CROMPTON, T. R.
Chemical Analysis of Additives in Plastics

ADDITIVE MIGRATION
FROM PLASTICS INTO FOOD

By

T. R. CROMPTON
M.Sc., F.R.I.C., M.Anal.Chem.

PERGAMON PRESS

OXFORD · NEW YORK · TORONTO · SYDNEY · PARIS · FRANKFURT

U.K.	Pergamon Press Ltd., Headington Hill Hall, Oxford OX3 0BW, England
U.S.A.	Pergamon Press Inc., Maxwell House, Fairview Park, Elmsford, New York 10523, U.S.A.
CANADA	Pergamon of Canada, Suite 104, 150 Consumers Road, Willowdale, Ontario M2J 1P9, Canada
AUSTRALIA	Pergamon Press (Aust.) Pty. Ltd., P.O. Box 544, Potts Point, N.S.W. 2011, Australia
FRANCE	Pergamon Press SARL, 24 rue des Ecoles, 75240 Paris, Cedex 05, France
FEDERAL REPUBLIC OF GERMANY	Pergamon Press GmbH, 6242 Kronberg-Taunus, Pferdstrasse 1, Federal Republic of Germany

First edition 1979

British Library Cataloguing in Publication Data
Crompton, Thomas Roy
Additive migration from plastics into food.
1. Food contamination 2. Plastics in
packaging 3. Plastics - Additives 4. Food
- Analysis
I. Title
614.3'1   TX571.P/   79-41018
ISBN 0-08-022465-2

In order to make this volume available as economically and as rapidly as possible the author's typescript has been reproduced in its original form. This method has its typographical limitations but it is hoped that they in no way distract the reader.

*Printed and bound in Great Britain by
William Clowes (Beccles) Limited, Beccles and London*

Contents

Preface

Plastics are now being used on a large scale for the packaging of foodstuffs and beverages, both non-alcoholic and alcoholic. This is evident for all to see on the supermarket shelf, viz. margerine packed in polystyrene tubs, wine and beer in PVC bottles and bacon in polyolefin shrunk wrap film. As well as at the point of sale, foods are increasingly shipped in bulk in plastic containers. Additionally there is the area of the increasing use of plastic utensils and containers in both the home and during the bulk preparation of food in restaurants, canteens, and food factories.

Where direct contact occurs between the packed commodity and the plastic it is likely that some transfer will occur of polymer additives, adventicious impurities such as monomers, catalyst remnants and residual polymerisation solvents and of low molecular weight polymer fractions from the plastic into the packaged material with the consequent risk of a toxic hazard to the consumer. The actual hazard arising to the consumer from any extractable material present is a function of two properties, namely the intrinsic toxicity of the neat extracted material as evaluated in animal feeding trials (not dealt with in this book) and the amount of the extracted material from the polymer which enters the packed food under service conditions, i.e. during the packaging operation and during the shelf life of the food to the time of consumption.

Most countries now have regulations regarding which polymer additives it is permitted and which it is not permitted to use in plastics which come into contact with foods, and indeed which it is permitted to use as a preservative in the food itself, and also for the permitted additives and other extractable substances present in polymers, regulations exist in many countries for the maximum amounts of these that shall migrate into the food under standardized test conditions.

As well as the foods themselves, many authorities have adopted various standard extraction liquids selected to simulate the action of actual foods for use in polymer extraction tests. The legal requirements concerning the use of additives in plastics in various countries are discussed in the final Chapter of the book.

To the analyst, the analysis of foods, beverages or simulent liquids which have been contacted with plastics either in extraction tests or during the shelf life of a packaged commodity, presents many fascinating and all too often difficult problems. Thus, the substance to be determined usually occurs at very low concentrations, several extracted substances may occur in the same food or simulent. For example the extract of a polystyrene may contain an antioxidant, an ultraviolet stabilizer

and antistatic agent, mineral oil and a plasticizer. Although the analyst may not
have to determine all of these, he will certainly have to be aware of any
interference effects that all these substances might have in the determination of
any particular component which he is interested in determining. Also, there is
the question of additive breakdown either during polymer manufacture or upon contact
with the food or simulent. Here there are two considerations, possible
interference effects of breakdown products on the determination of the additive
and the necessity, often, to identify and determine the breakdown product as it
in itself must be considered from the toxicity point of view.

The solution of such problems requires the full range of modern analytical
technology now available to the chemist .

The first two Chapters of the book discuss, respectively, the various types of
plastics, used in food packaging and the types of substances present in the plastic,
whether deliberately added or not which might migrate into the food.

The remainder of the book reviews for the first time world literature on the
subject covering extraction testing and the analysis of extractants. Much
previously unpublished material is included. It is hoped that the inclusion, in
some instances, of detailed examples of food extractant analysis will be of
assistance to workers in the field and will assist them in developing
modifications of these procedures to suit their particular problems.

In addition to the direct technique of analysing foods and simulent liquids for
extracted polymer components which is the technique normally used, and the one
which is discussed in this book, there does exist another method of approach to
the analysis which involves determining the migrating polymer component in the
polymer both before and after contact with the food or the simulent extraction
liquid, the decrease in concentration in the polymer gives an estimate of the
amount which has entered the food or extractant. This enters the field of
analysis of additives in polymers and the authors recently revised book "Chemical
Analysis of Additives in Plastics" Pergamon 2nd edition (1977) will be found
very useful in this respect.

The latter book is also recommended to those who wish to ascertain which additives
and other substances are present in a polymer in order to decide on which
particular substances to look for in extraction liquids obtained in extraction
tests.

The book will be of interest to anyone in the plastics industry concerned with
the manufacture of foodstuff or beverage grades of polymers and to those in the
food and beverage packaging industry who use such plastics for packaging, also to
large retail outlets such as supermarkets who wish to evaluate the safety aspects
of packagings they adopt.

Workers in other industries which use plastics in applications which involve
contact between the plastic and substances which either internally or externally
contact the human body (pharmaceuticals and cosmetics) will find much to interest
them.

The book will also be of interest to our legislators who are concerned with
formulating regulations concerning the packaging in plastics and to medical and
public health authorities who are concerned with the effects of what we eat and
drink on our health.

Finally, as a branch of environmental science, it is hoped that the contents of
the book will be of interest to environmentalists who are concerned with the

effects of the intrusion of foreign chemicals via our food on the quality of life and also to those members of the general public, who, increasingly, are taking an interest in such topics.

Acknowledgements

The author acknowledges with thanks, permission to reproduce figures given by the publishers of the following journals:

La Chimia e l'Industria - Figs. 1-6.

Analyst (London) - Figs. 20-22, Table 24.

Food and Cosmetic Technology - Figs. 24-28, 48-52, 61-63, Tables 27-30, 32-35, 37-39.

Deutsch Lebensmittel Rundschau - Figs. 29-33, 47, 53-57, 60, Tables 31, 36.

Fette Seifen Anstrichmittel - Figs. 64-66, Table 40.

Chapter 1

Types of Polymers Used in Food Packaging

A high proportion of the wide range of polymers manufactured nowadays are used in applications which involve contact with food or beverages particularly in foodstuff packaging applications, utensils, kitchenware and in processing equipment in food factories and other establishments where food is handled in large quantities. In addition to packaging applications, plastics are used extensively in the food and drink vending market and in the manufacture of prepacked meals.

In this Chapter the types of plastics that are being used in these applications are briefly reviewed. The variants of these polymers such as copolymers and blends are discussed together with a brief general discussion of the properties of the polymers which are most relevant from the point of view of their use in applications involving contact with food.

Polyolefins

Polyethylene

There are two distinct forms of polyethylene, namely low density (high pressure synthesis) and high density (low pressure synthesis e.g. the Ziegler Route). Also available are a range of copolymers of intermediate density made by either blending or by the copolymerization of ethylene with other olefins such as propene, butane or hexene. The density range for polymers produced by the low pressure route is about 0.945 to 0.965 g/cm^3, whereas the high pressure process produces material with densities between 0.918 and 0.935 g/cm^3. Crystallinities are also different for the two types of polyethylene. The high density polyethylene with its linear structure favours parallel configuration of the chains and hence a high degree of crystallinity (75-90%). The low density polyethylene has appreciable chain branching which disturbs the regularity of the arrangement of atoms and hence produces a low degree of crystallinity (55-70%). The greater linearity of high density polyethylene also increases the softening point of this grade relative to that of low density polyethylenes. This in turn increases the flex resistance of the high density polymer. Due to its high softening point, high density polyethylene unlike the low density variety can be steam sterilized, a property which is of importance in the food packaging field. Both forms of polyethylene are fairly inert chemically and are not attacked by solvents at temperatures up to 60°C. However, they do absorb certain hydrocarbon solvents with swelling at room temperature. The high density polymer is more resistant in this respect. Both polymers are resistant to water and salt solutions and water absorption is negligible at room temperature. Water vapour permeability is fairly low in

1

the high density polymer, as would be expected having the lower permeability. Gas
permeabilities are not particularly low, and low density polyethylene, in
particular, is not to be recommended as an oxygen barrier, i.e. would not be used
for the packaging of types of foods where oxygen ingress is undesirable. Water
and oxygen permeabilities have important implications in the consideration of these
polymers as food packaging materials.

Both high and low density polyethylenes exhibit the phenomenon of environmental
stress cracking. This can occur when the material is multiaxially stressed when
in contact with certain polar liquids or vapours. These liquids need not be
solvents for polyethylene or even be more than slightly absorbed by it, and if
the polymer is unstrained (i.e. no moulding strains) no cracking occurs, no
matter how long the contact time with the liquids. Environmental stress cracking
has implications in the food packaging field as certain foodstuffs, such as
vegetable oils and alcoholic beverages can act as stress cracking agents.

Various types of additives can occur in polyethylene used in food packaging.
These include, pigments, carbon black (for ultraviolet light resistance), slip
additives (e.g. silica) to lower coefficient of friction of film and improve the
rate of movement of film through printing and wrapping equipment, antistatic
additives (to reduce dust attraction caused by build up of static changes),
antiblock additives (used in film grades used for making bags in order to overcome difficulties in separating them from a pile) also to facilitate rapid
opening of the bags on automatic filling equipment, antioxidants (to prevent
degradation during processing and during service life of the article). These and
other types of additives and adventicious non-polymer components which occur in
polyethylenes are discussed in more detail in Chapter 2.

Uses of polyolefins

In this Chapter the discussion on the uses of the polymers is limited to their
applications in the polymers that in any way come into contact with food or
beverages. The biggest single application for low density polyethylene is in
packaging. Food contact applications include the household use of polyethylene
bags for storing food, especially in the refridgerator, or freezer, polyethylene
coated cartons for frozen foods, bags for pre-packed fresh produce and bags for
frozen poultry and hams. Blow moulded polyethylene containers are used for the
packaging of table salt and sauces. In the injection moulding field, however,
low and high density polyethylene are used in many types of food containers,
particularly as closures and dispensers. Another very large use is in pots,
tubs, beakers and bowls used as food storage containers. There is also an
increasing use of extruded low density polyethylene pipe for domestic cold water
supplies.

Polypropylene

Polypropylene manufactured by the low pressure route gives a polymer which is
largely isotactic (pendant methyl groups all on same side of carbon backbone).
The crystallinity of low pressure polypropylene at 65 to 70% is somewhat lower
than that of high density polyethylene.

Polypropylene, unlike the polyethylenes, is not subject to environmental stress
cracking, which gives it an advantage in the food packaging field. It also has a
lower density $(0.90g/cm^3)$ than either low or high density polyethylene. Although
the impact strength of polypropylene is lower than that of high density polyethylene, especially at temperatures below 0^oC, this can be improved by
incorporating into polypropylene various synthetic rubbers or by copolymerization
with ethylene and propylene.

Two important properties of polypropylene are its resiliance and its resistance
to fatigue by flexing. This makes it a suitable material for moulding
screw cap closures used extensively in food and beverage packaging. A thin
section diaphragm or fin is moulded into the inner surface of the closure in
such a position that it bears down on the upper surface of the bottle neck. A
rigid material would not have enough "give" to take up imperfections in the glass
surface and so would not form as good a seal. On the other hand, a more flexible
material, such as low density polyethylene, would "give" but would not press back
strongly enough to form a seal. The good fatigue resistance of popypropylene is
utilized in the manufacture of snap fit lid food containers.

Injection moulded polypropylene is used extensively in the manufacture of food
storage containers either thick walled or thin walled. Polypropylene, due to its
higher softening point when compared to polyethylene, is useful in food packaging
applications where hot filling temperatures are involved. Polypropylene film is
used extensively in food packaging applications because of its low water vapour
and oxygen permeabilities. Examples include, biscuits, potato crisps and snack
foods. Animal feeding stuffs are packed in polypropylene woven sacks, as are
grains, sugar and vegetables.

Poly (4 - methyl pentene - 1) TPX

This is a polymer of 4-methylpentene -1. It is a low specific gravity (0.83 g/cm^3)
polymer of high clarity and softening point. It is still rather expensive. It
has a lower impact strength and a very much higher permeability to gas and water
vapour than either polyethylene or polypropylene. It is highly resistant to
aqueous salt solutions, acids, alkalies and organic solvents. It is subject to
environmental stress cracking.

One of its few applications in which it comes into contact with food is as a
coating on trays used in bakery ovens. In general its outstanding properties
compared to the other polyolefins are resistance to hot filling and outstanding
clarity.

Ethylene - vinyl acetate copolymers

These polymers are very similar to low density polyethylene in many of their
characteristics. They are more transparent than polyethylene and have a high
flexibility and impact resistance and good resilience. These polymers have a
high permeability to water vapour and gases and are rather more susceptable to
oil/hydrocarbon attack than is low density polyethylene. When made into film,
ethylene - vinyl acetate has a greater tendency towards blocking than low density
polyethylene and consequently it is necessary to incorporate a rather high
percentage of antiblocking additive. Applications are mainly in the fields where
flexibility and resilience are useful, particularly at low temperatures. This
makes these copolymers attractive, for example, for the stretch wrapping of deep
forzen poultry in which application they require a close contour wrap of the bird.

Ionomers

The only ionomer which is at present produced in commercial quantities is
manufactured by Dupont under the trade name of Surlyn A. Ionomers are, in effect,
ionic polymers which are solid at normal temperatures but which soften as do
thermoplastics upon heating. Surlyn A is basically a polymer of ethylene
containing carboxylate groups and which is similar in many ways to low density
polythene. The ionic forces, due to the carboxylate groups give it a high melt
strength so that it has excellent drawing characteristics. Surlyn A is useful as
an extrusion material and very thin coatings with a low 'neck -in' can be obtained.
Skin packaging is another application with obvious attractions in the food

packaging industry. It is resistant to strong and weak alkalies and is slowly
attacked by acids. It is resistant to alcohol but swells in contact with oils and
hydrocarbons. It is, however, more resistant to oils than low density polyethylene
and has in fact been used for the packaging of olive oil.

Vinyl plastics and vinyl copolymers

Polyvinyl chloride is much less crystalline than the polyolefins. The base
polymer is very hard and for most applications is has to be plasticised to make it
flexible enough for use. There are many plasticisers available for PVC. Food
contact applications, of course, impose their own requirements of intrinsic safety
and low migration rate of the plasticiser. Due to the nearness of its decomposition
and processing temperatures PVC has to be stabilized against heat by the addition
of 1-2% of heat stabilizer and this, in turn, has food contact implications.

PVC has a density of about 1.4 g/cm^3 which makes it appreciably denser than any of
the unchlorinated polyolefins. It is resistant to alcohol and to many fats and
this leads to its applications in the packaging of wine, beer, and fatty foods.

For food contact uses PVC usually has a low plasticiser content in which form it
has good rigidity and can be moulded into sections and film down to 75 mm thick.
It has the merit of clarity, which is useful in many food uses.

PVC film can be thermoformed into various packages including tubs, trays for
foodstuffs, inserts for chocolate boxes and biscuit tins and other confectioneries.
Very thin film is used for shrink wrapping of prepackaged meat, fruit and
vegetables. PVC bottles are increasingly being used for the packing of foodstuffs
and alcoholic beverages, including wine and beer. It is used extensively in U.K.
for the packaging of fruit squashes and to some extent for edible cooking oils.
PVC can be fabricated into jars suitable for the packaging of coffee and
chocolate drinks.

PVC is also copolymerized with other monomers such as vinyl acetate, vinylidene
chloride propylene and acrylonitrile. Copolymerization with vinyl acetate tends
to soften the polymer to the point that plasticiser addition may be unnecessary.
For low temperature applications, plasticiser addition may still be desirable and
in this form the copolymer finds application in the fabrication of refrigerator
trays.

Vinyl chloride - vinylidene chloride copolymers are used for the manufacture of
films which have a very low permeability to water vapour and gases. Such film is
used for wrapping cheese and other commodities which require the absence of
oxygen for their preservation.

Vinyl chloride - vinylidene chloride is also applied as a coating to improve the
barrier properties of other food packaging materials such as paper, polypropylene
and cellulose film.

Propylene - vinyl chloride copolymers are used mainly as bottle blowing materials.
Copolymers of vinyl chloride and acrylonitrile have no food packaging applications.

Polyvinyl acetate

This polymer is used in the food industry, mainly as an adhesive particularly in
laminating operations.

Polystyrene and its copolymers

This is a hard fairly brittle material. Chemically it is unaffected by acids, alkalies, lower alcohols and most paraffinic hydrocarbons. It is attacked by certain foodstuffs e.g. orange peel oil. It is a reasonably good barrier to gas but a poor one to water vapour.

The brittleness of polystyrene can be overcome by incorporation of a synthetic rubber, such as polybutadiene or styrene-butadiene rubber in amounts up to 10%. The increase in impact strength and flexibility thus acquired is accompanied by some loss in clarity, so that only opaque or translucent grades of toughened polystyrene are available. This does not however, limit its uses in food packaging.

Polystyrene is also available in an expanded (cellular) form and as such finds extensive application in the fabrication of drink vending machine cups.

Polystyrene is used extensively in food packaging and in the home. The toughened polymer is injection moulded into tubs and containers for yogurt, dairy cream, cut peel, ice cream, cottage cheese, honey and syrup. Transparant untoughened polystyrene is used for the fabrication of jam and marmalade containers. Thermo-formed thin section toughened polystyrene is used for the fabrication of vending cups, and thicker sections are used to manufacture refrigerator cabinets and door liners where food contact is likely. Bioxially orientated untoughened polystyrene film is also used in the manufacture of transparent food containers. Moulded expanded polystyrene boxes are used extensively for the transport of fruit, vegetables and fish and thermoformed expanded sheet to produce supermarket trays for the prepackaging of meat, fruit and vegetables.

The physical properties of polystyrene are improved by copolymerisation with acryonitrile or acrylonitrile and butadiene. Styrene – acrylonitrile (SAN) is tough and transparent and finds application in the manufacture of measuring jugs, orange and lemon squeezers and food homogenizers.

Acrylonitrile-butadiene – styrene (ABS) can be manufactured to have a range of properties, depending on the ratio of the monomers present and the order in which the monomers are polymerized.

ABS has an improved impact resistance and toughness over polystyrene and also superior chemical resistance. It can be injection moulded, blow moulded and extruded. Applications in food packaging include injection moulded cake and bread trays and margarine tubs.

Acrylics

Polymethylmethacrylate.

This is a very clear plastic with good light exposure properties. Chemically it is resistant to water, alkalies, many dilute acids and aqueous salt solutions. This polymer is too expensive for packaging. It does however have one application as a food quality plastic, namely the fabrication of artificial dentures.

Polyacrylonitrile.

This polymer has good chemical and oil and grease resistance. Its only application in which it might come into contact with food is as a filter cloth in food manufacturing equipment.

XT Polymer.

This is a copolymer of acrylic acid and two other monomers. It has excellent oil and grease resistance and has, in fact been used for the fabrication of containers for peanut butter and medicinal mineral oil.

Lopac

This is the trade name for a copolymer of methacrylonitrile with small percentages of styrene and methyl styrene.

It is at present a development product but it may have possible future application as a material for the fabrication of carbonated soft drink bottles. It has excellent clarity and barrier properties.

Borex

This is the trade name of a product made by copolymerising acrylonitrile and methyl acrylate in the presence of butadiene - acrylonitrile rubber. It is clear, has good barrier properties and impact strength. This polymer, also, may have future applications in the bottle blowing field for carbonated soft drinks.

Fluorocarbon polymers

Due to its chemical inertness polyterafluoroethylene is used for pump and pipe lining and, as such, may be used in applications which involve contact with food. In addition, it is used as a non-stick coating in pans and frying pans and is used in the food industry for the coating of a wide range of mixing equipment. Due to its high price, this material would not find application as a food packaging material.

Nylons (polyamides)

Various nylons are manufactured by the condensation of amino acids. Nylons can be blown into film and here they find many applications in the packaging of oils, fats and greases. The high softening point of nylons have lead to their extensive use in boil-in the bag food packs. The low gas permeability of the film has been utilized in sachets for vacuum packed foods, such as cheese slices and bacon. Moulded articles in nylon are widely used in food manufacturing processes. The fact that Nylons are self lubricating and consequently do not require the addition of a lubricant additive is a particularly important factor in the food industry where contamination by lubricants cannot be tolerated.

Polyethylene terephthalate (Terylene)

This is a condensation product of ethylene glycol and terephthalic acid. It is fabricated as film and fibre and can be injection moulded. Terylene film has excellent strength and transparency but tends to lose strength at the heat seals. Bags are, therefore, often made up using adhesives. It has a high softening point. As a moulded material its important properties are low moisture pick-up, high yield strength and high surface hardness. It has good creep and abrasion resistance.

Terylene film is used mainly in the manufacture of food packaging. It is expensive but due to its high strength, it can be used as a very thin film which keeps costs down. When used as a thin film it is sometimes laminated with other lower cost film. Its high softening point renders it attractive in the boil-in-the-bag food market.

Polycarbonates,

These polymers are, in effect, linear polyesters of carbonic acid made by reacting aromatic dehydroxy compounds such as Bisphenol A with diphenylcarbonate or phosgene.

Polycarbonates are hard, rigid and transparent with a very high impact and tensile strength. They have good low temperature properties and are resistant to acids but not alkalies. Polycarbonates are stain resistant and have been found to be satisfactory after long periods in contact with coffee, fruit juices and tea. An additional bonus with this material is its non-flammability.

Because of its high stain resistance, high temperature resistance and impact strength, this polymer is used for the fabrication of household items such as plates, cups and saucers and babies feeding bottles. It has also found some application in the fabrication of food processing equipment.

Polyacetals

Polyacetal homopolymer is essentially a polymer of formaldehyde. Copolymers with cyclic ethers, such as ethylene oxide are also available commercially.

These polymers have good abrasion resistance and stand up well to repeated impacts. The range of applicability extends from -40°C to 80°C. They have a low water absorption and are creep and fatigue resistant. Chemically they are very resistant to weak and strong alkalies and detergents but are attacked by strong acids. They are affected by ultraviolet light but can be protected with carbon black. The properties of polyacetal have lead to a particular specialised food contact application such as the meat hooks for handling carcass meat.

Polyphenylene oxide (PPO)

This is a linear polymer made by the catalytic oxidative coupling of 2,6 dimethyl-phenol. PPO has a use temperature range of -55 to 175°C. It is transparent but yellow in colour and is rather expensive being used mainly in engineering applications. Its resistance to repeated steam sterilizations makes it a useful plastic in food engineering applications. It is also used in the fabrication of domestic food mixers.

A modified form of PPO is available with the trade name Noryl (General Electric Company). This is cheaper than PPO and has excellent mechanical properties over the range -40 to 120°C. This polymer is used extensively in food contact applications where an impact strength slightly inferior to that of PPO is acceptable.

Polysulphone

This is another engineering plastic used in food engineering. It is a tough rigid transparent plastic with very high tensile strength, creep resistance and low mould shrinkage and water absorption. It is resistant to acids, alkalies, acqueous salt solutions, alcohols, detergents and oils even at elevated temperatures and under moderate stress. It has also been used in kitchen hardware and as a replacement for stainless steel in the manufacture of milking machines.

Thermosets

Various thermosets are used in contact with food in significant commercial amounts. Thermosets are distinguished from thermoplastics in that they undergo an irreversible chemical change on heating during moulding. Thermosets are discussed below.

Phenol Formaldehyde

As manufactured, these polymers usually contain various types of fillers and this has obvious food contact implications. The fillers are used to reduce cost, improve shock resistance and to reduce mould shrinkage. Phenol-formaldehyde resins are resistant to common solvents, acids, aqueous salt solutions and hot oils, although water and alcohols cause slight swelling. As far as food contact applications are concerned the main use of these resins is in the manufacture of closures for containers such as jars and bottles. Direct contact is less likely in these applications because of the interposition of a liner between the closure and the container. The resins are also used for moulding the handles of kitchen implements.

Urea formaldehyde

This resin produces mouldings which are resistant to common solvents but are attacked by strong acids. This resin is slightly less resistant to water than phenol-formaldehyde. The impact strength of urea-formaldehyde resins depend on the type of filler used. Frequently, bleached wood pulp is used as a filler. The main interest to the food industry is again that of container closured and in the domestic field they are used as casings for domestic food mixers.

Melamine - formaldehyde

Colourless white or pastel coloured mouldings can be produced from this resin using bleached wood pulp as a filler. Melamine-formaldehyde mouldings are more resistant to water than urea-formaldehyde resins and are not attacked by weak alkalies and have a high heat resistance.

Due to their superior water resistance, mouldings made in this resin have good staining resistance and have consequently been widely used in tableware. Their high heat resistance has lead to their extensive use as the top layer of decorative laminates for table tops and working surfaces.

Polyesters

A whole range of these resins is available. They are produced by the reaction of polyhydric alcohols and polybasic acids. An important use of these resins is in the manufacture of glass fibre reinforced polyester laminates which, in addition to their great strength have a high heat and corrosion resistance.

Thermosetting polyesters are resistant to most solvents and acids and alkalies. Glass reinforced plastics are widely used in the manufacture of semi bulk containers for all types of liquid and solids and for storage tanks.

Epoxy resins

This range of resins, made by the condensation of Bisphenol A and epichlorhydrin or another compound containing the epoxy group have many similarities with the polyesters. These are extremely tough materials with good heat and chemical resistance. They have low impact strength and when used as coatings are usually modified with flexibilising agents such as low molecular weight Nylons.

Epoxy resins, as polyesters, are used in the manufacture of laminates and reinforced structures. They are used as lacquers in a wide variety of food cans.

Polyurethanes

These resins are formed by the reaction of isocyanates such as toluene di iso-cyanate and methylene di isocyanate with polyols. This resin can be produced in a rigid form or as a rigid or flexible foam. Applications of polyurethane foam in food packaging are likely to be confined to cushioning, for example, glass jars in outer containers, since polyurethanes must not be used in contact with food because of the great difficulty in removing the last traces of the di-isocyanate which is highly toxic.

Silicones

There are three main forms of silicones, namely liquids, solids (resins) and rubbers. The resins are the most important from the food contact point of view. A major application is in the bakery industry where the resin is used to coat bread baking tins.

Natural polymers

Various natural materials such as cellulose and cellulose acetate are used in applications which involve contact with food. These are discussed below.

Cellulose

Cellulose film is manufactured by a rather complicated process involving the casting of the film and impregnation with plasticisers and flexibilisers such as glycerol or ethylene glycol to produce uncoated film which is non-moistureproof and non-heat sealable. To make it moisture-proof and heat sealable a coating of nitrocellulose is applied. To obtain a superior moisture barrier a coating of vinyl chloride - vinylidene copolymer (Saran) is applied. A wide variety of grades of such film are manufactured. There are many possible variations with regenerated cellulose film. These include various degrees of moisture-proofness and single sided coatings. Variants which are in regular production include the following types, nitrocellulose coated on both sides (moisture-proof), heat sealable, non moisture-proof, nitrocellulose coated on one side only and copolymer coated on both sides.

Regenerated cellulose film has a light transmission equal to that of glass. Dry cellulose film is practically impermeable to the permanent gases but necomes permeable when wet. Moisture vapour permeability is very high unless the film is coated.

Both moisture-proof and non-moistureproof film have a wide variety of uses including important applications in the food packaging field. Non-moistureproof films are used when protection from grease and dirt is required but where mould growth would be a problem if a good moisture barrier were used, examples of its use in this area include packaging of meat pies, cakes, fondants, chocolate coated sweets and fresh sausages. Moistureproof films are used for the wrapping of hygroscopic foodstuffs such as biscuits, sugar, confectionary, potato crisps, bread and shelled nuts. Moistureproof film is also used for the packaging of hygroscopic sweets and of pharmaceuticals and dried milk.

Single side coated film is used for the packaging of fresh meat with the uncoated side in contact with the meat. The moistening of the film by the meat raises its permeability to gases including oxygen and so gives it the right combination of conditions to preserve the fresh colour of the meat. A single coated film is also used when extrusion coating with polyethylene is required. The polyethylene readily adheres more securely to the base cellulose film than to the nitrocellulose coating. This type of laminate is used for the vacuum packing of bacon, cheese and coffee.

Cellulose derivitives

Cellulose tri-acetate and diacetate (secondary cellulose acetate).
This is a hard tough material made by the acetylation of cellulose. It is sensitive to moisture pickup and is dimensionally unstable. It is resistant to weak acids

and alkalies but is decomposed by strong ones. Both the triacetate and the
secondary cellulose acetate give crystal clear films with high gas and water vapour
permeabilities.

Cellulose triacetate finds limited use in applications involving contact with food,
(cutlery handles). The secondary acetate film is widely used in packaging,
principally as a laminate. It is not readily heat sealed. It does, however,
readily accept printing inks. Cellulose secondary acetate is normally used as the
outer layer of a laminate with an inner heat sealable coating. Printing is carried
out on the inside of the acetate thus giving a glossy decoration. Secondary
acetate film is also used as the window in cartons as it has good adhesion to
cardboard. The high permeability of cellulose acetate film to water vapour and
oxygen limits its uses in fresh food packaging. It is, however, particularly useful if a breathable film is required allowing the inward passage of carbon
dioxide. This renders it particularly useful in certain specific food packaging
applications.

Thicker section secondary acetate film is used for the manufacture of rigid food
containers and vacuum drawn cellulose acetate containers are used in packaging
sweets and chocolates at the high price end of the market.

Ethyl cellulose

This is manufactured by reacting cellulose with ethyl chloride. It is tough and
retains flexibility and impact strength down to $-40^{\circ}C$ and has a similar moisture
pickup to cellulose acetate. It is widely used as a moulding material and in
film manufacture.

Chapter 2

Non-Plastics Components of Plastics

All polymers, in addition to the basic plastic, contain usually several, if not a multiplicity of non-polymeric components in amounts from less than one part per millom to several percents. These substances obviously have implications in the suitabilities or otherwise of the plastic for applications involving contact with foodstuffs. Thus, although the plastic itself, due to its very high molecular weight, might not contaminate the foodstuff it is apparent that certain of the additives, which are usually of relatively low molecular weight and therefore of higher solubility will be transferred from the plastic to the foodstuff during storage. This raises questions regarding the toxicity of the additives, the amounts which transfer and the possible implications of this, from the toxicity point of view, as far as the food consumer is concerned.

Non-polymeric components are present in plastics either unavoidably as a result of the process of manufacture or as the result of deliberate additions to the plastic in order to improve some aspect of ease of manufacture or final polymer properties.

Thus non-polymeric components can be subdivided into three groups:

> Polymerisation residues
> Processing aids
> End-product additives

Polymerisation residues cover substances whose presence is to a large extent unavoidable such as low molecular weight polymer oligomers catalyst remnants, polymerisation solvents. Raw material non-polymerisable impurities and impurities picked up from plant materials. Processing aids include such substances as thermal antioxidants and heat stabilizers added to prevent decomposition of the polymer during moulding and slip additives to facilitate moulding. The third group again are deliberately added to the polymer either during manufacture or subsequently to improve the properties of the final polymer. As discussed below, a very wide range of non-polymeric substances are used in this category ranging from secondary thermal antioxidant to impact improvers, plasticisers, ultra-violet stabilisers, antistatic agents etc.

The situation regarding the presence of non-polymeric low molecular weight additives in polymers can be best illustrated by an actual example concerning a batch of polypropylene which, upon detailed but by no means complete examination, was shown to contain the constituents listed below. In many instances the probably origin of these substances can be ascribed. Thus, in this single polymer

substances falling under the three catagories previously mentioned were found.
These include Ziegler catalyst remnants, neutralising chemicals, residual monomer
and polymerisation solvent (polymerisation residues), a calcium salt and an anti-
oxidant(processing aids) and a further antioxidant a light stabilizer and a filler
(end product additives).

Non Polymeric Components found in a sample of Polypropylene

determined	concentration ppm	origin
polymerisation residues		
aluminium	40	remnants of Ziegler
titanium	5	organoaluminium-
chlorine	230	titanium halide catalysts
sodium	30	catalyst neutralisation
potassium	18	alkalies
silicon	<20	general
iron	5	contamination
manganese	0.1	from plant
nickel	8	
tin	0.3	
vanadium	<0.2	
zinc	<10	
chromium	1	
C_6/C_{16} hydrocarbons	900	unreacted monomer
dissolved propylene	1 cc/cc polymer	residual polymerisation solvent
Processing aids		
calcium	40	possibly calcium stearote stabilizer for protecting polymer during moulding
Ionol	200	antioxidant (thermally degraded Ionol also present)
End product additives		
barium	1000	possible barium sulphate filler
substituted benzopheno (2-hydroxy 4 n-octoxybenzophenone)		light stabiliser
dilaurythiodipropionate ppm sulphur found)		'probable secondary antioxidant.

Further information on the various types of non-polymeric components that can occur
in polymers is discussed below under separate headings. This information will be
of assistance to the chemist in enabling him to select the types of components to
expect in various types of polymers used in food manufacture.

Polymerisation Residues

Low pressure polyethylene might contain minute traces of oxygen or nitrogen or sulphur chain transfer catalyst residues. These are usually labile and can be ignored from the foodstuff contamination point of view. Polymers such as poly- ethylene, polypropylene and polystyrene manufactured by a catalysed low pressure route will however, usually contain appreciable catalyst residues usually appearing in the form of titanium, aluminium, magnesium and chromium, also possibly lithium and sodium. As the example quoted earlier indicates these impurities can occur in the polymer at levels approaching 100ppm.

Suspension or emulsion processes for the polymerisation of styrene or vinyl chloride can impart to the polymer significant amounts (up to 0.05%) of proton donating processing chemicals such as potassium and ammonium persulphate or benzyl and lauryl peroxide and their decomposition products, (respectively potassium sulphate, ammonium carbonate, urea and benzoic or lauric acid) and these are of significance in relation to safety in use for food.

Catalysts and accelerators used in the manufacture of thermosets include peroxides, organic nitrogen compounds and copper and cobalt salts of napthenic and other organic acids.

Residual and Unreacted Starting Materials

Many manufactured polymers contain either unreacted monomer, or low molecular weight polymer (oligomers) in amounts varying from a few parts per million to several per cent depending on the manufacturing process used and the type of polymer. Low molecular weight products are particularly prevelent in thermosets. However, even polymers such as polyethylene contain a small amount (usually less than 1%) of a waxy low molecular weight tail, whose solubility characteristics and therefore extactability into foods is different from that of the main polymer product. Low pressure polyolefins in fact can contain up to 1% on a volume - volume basis of unreacted monomer, especially when the polymer is newly manufactured.

Simple monomers, such as styrene, ethylene, propylene, hexene, vinyl chloride, acrylonitrile and caprolactam,   indeed, usually do occur in the corresponding polymers. In addition to unreacted monomer, any non-polymerisable impurities in the original monomer feed to the polymerisation could occur in the final product. Thus, styrene monomer can contain low concentrations of numerous saturated and unsaturated hydrocarbons, ethyl benzene being particularly prevelent and these, particularly the saturated compounds which do not polymerise, will occur in the finished polymer and have implications in the use of the polymer food packaging. It is not unknown for compounds as toxic as benzene to occur at very low concentrations, usually less than 10 parts per million in styrene monomer, and this could, therefore, also occur in the polymer. For foodgrades of polystyrene, the monomer content is usually nowadays limited to 0.2% maximum. Acrylonitrile monomer may be found in amounts up to 0.1% in finished polymer, whilst negligible amounts of monomer are found in Nylon and poly-4-methyl-pentene-1. With thermosets, phenol and formaldelyde are likely to be found even in the most carefully manufactured grades.

Regarding oligomers, only those in the relatively very low molecular weight range, and these are usually only greases, are of sufficient potential significance to be regarded as non-polymeric impurities, which may have foodstuff packaging implications. Thus, polypropylene may contain traces of dimer (C_6H_{12}) and tetramer ($C_{12}H_{24}$), hydrocarbons with molecular weight up to approximately 200. The full chemistry of the low molecular weight tail composition, has not yet been fully studied in the case of many polymer systems, especially in the case of copolymers involving two or more monomers.

Polymerisation Medium

Particularly in the case of Ziegler-Natta type low pressure polymerisations of olefins, the reaction is usually performed in an inert paraffinic solvent medium (from C_4 to C_{18}). In such cases, of course, traces of this solvent are found in the final polymer which persist for a long time and, indeed, are difficult to remove even by treatment of the polymer in vacuum.

In the case of polystyrene and polyvinyl chloride, made by the suspension or emulsion processes, the reaction medium is an aqueous solution containing wetting agents, detergents, soaps and emulsifiers. Traces of all of these will occur in the final product.

Catalyst Decomposition Agents

Upon completion of the polymerisation of polyolefins by the Ziegler-Nutta low pressure routine, the organo-aluminium-titanium halide catalyst is decomposed and neutralized by the addition of low molecule weight alcohols and possibly aqueous wetting agents and soaps whilst pH control may be effected by the addition of aqueous alkalies such as sodium carbonate. This stage of the process can therefore introduce alcohols and alkali metal salts into the polymer.

Other impurities introduced during polymerisation

These include general contamination from plant materials such as iron, silica, copper, oil, etc.

Further sources of contamination include polymerisation inhibitors (styrene and vinyl chloride monomers), emulsifying, suspension and chain transfer agents (polystyrene, polyvinyl chloride).

Chemicals Added During Polymerisation

In this category is included the addition of up to 10% mineral oil (to impart flexibility to the product during the manufacture of high impact polystyrene by the copolymerisation of styrene and synthetic rubbers).

Processing Aids

The main types of processing aids are discussed below under separate headings:

          Antiblock agents
          Antioxidants
          Antisplit Agents
          Antistatic agents
          Heat stabilisers
          Lubricants
          Melt strength improvers
          Mould release agents
          Plasticisers
          Slip additives
          Other stabilisers

Antiblock Agents. The principal antiblock agent used is silica at the 0.1 to 0.5%
level. Its function is to prevent sticking in thin films of the polymer.

Antioxidants. Antioxidants which prevent degradation of the polymer by reaction
with atmospheric oxygen may be required during moulding operations on the polymer
and will be needed to prevent oxygen pickup and oxidation and embrittlement of
polymer during long term usage. The reaction of polymers with oxygen are chain
reactions involving hydroperoxy radicals and these reactions can be inhibited or
slowed down by compounds known as antioxidants which interrupt the chain reaction
at some point. Typical antioxidants are notably hindered phenols and organic
sulphides.

Antisplit agents. These are used to prevent spontaneous fibrillation or oriented
polypropylene film in processing equipment. These additives are usually natural
or synthetic rubber added at concentrations up to 10%.

Antistatic agents. Plastics, being good electrical insulators retain electrostatic
changes developed by friction between the plastic itself, between plastic and
moving machinery, or by electroinisation from dust or radiation. These changes on
the plastic lead to end-use problems such as ticking of flowing polymer powders,
sticking together or polymer film and dust attraction with the development of a
dirty appearance. Also, discharges to earth can lead to the formation of pin-holes
in films and electric shocks to operators, fire hazards and explosions of stored
petroleum.

The requirements of an antistatic agent are a reasonable electrical conductivity
and an ability to migrate to the surface of the plastic moulding or film as it is
on the surface that the electrostatic charge concentrates.

The selection of the types of compounds used as antistatic additives is governed
by complex considerations, one of which is that it should have the correct degree
of compatability with the base polymer which will enable it to migrate to the
polymer surface at a controlled rate during service life.

The majority of antistatic agents now in use are either gly col derivatives or
quarternary ammonium salt derivatives. Lauric diethanolamide is a typical antistatic additive used in the formulation of polyolefins. The reasons for including
antistatic agents in a polymer formulation intended for food packaging are mainly
the avoidance of sticking together of films and thin plastic sections such as cups
during food packaging operations. Avoidance of dust attraction in film and mouldings
is a lesser problem in the case of food packaging dur to the relatively low interval
of time intervening between packaging and sale.

Heat stabilisers. These are incorporated into the polymer to protect it from
decomposition during the short time that it is held at a relatively high
temperature in the moulding machine. Low density polyethylene and nylons are
generally sufficiently stable not to require heat stabilisers. Polystyrene
requires slittle stabilisation and high density polyethylene, polypropylene and PVC
may require significant additions of such stabilisers. A wide range or heat
stabilisers are available and the choice is dictated by considerations of the
temperature to be encountered and the time at which the polymer is held at an
elevated temperature, also the presence of or absence of atmospheric oxygen and
of antioxidants.

Lubricants. Internal lubricants are used to reduce the viscosity of the molten
polymer in the extruder. These additives may be virtually any compatable stable
compound and include compounds such as plasticisers and C_{12} - C_{30} hydrocarbons
added at the several percent level.

External lubricants are used to reduce the friction between the polymer and the surface of the extruding equipment. To function effectively these should be not too soluble in the plastic in order to enhance the concentration of lubricant at the surface. The most commonly used external lubricant is calcium stearate added at the 0.05 to 0.3 per cent level.

Melt strength improvers. In extrusion blow moulding operations molten polymer passes through a stage where it is processed with little external support. In these circumstances the moulding is likely to distort. The incorporation of a melt strength additive reduces the possibility of this occuring. Frequently, the materials used to improve melt strength are the same as those used for internal lubrication or plasticisation.

Mould release agents. These are used to coat the mould in order to reduce the possibility that the moulded article will stick. Silicones are usually now used for this purpose, although paraffin oil or petroleum jelly are still used to a small extent.

Plasticisers. Almost any soluble organic compound can be used to plasticise a polymer including high boiling alcohol esters of phthalic, adipic, sebacic and phosporic acids and ethylene oxide condensates and polychlorinated hydrocarbons. Polymeric high molecular weight plasticisers are occasionally used. Due to their lower solubility in foods, the general tendency is for these to extract from plastics into food at a lower rate than non-polymeric plasticisers. Good compatability, low volatility, freedom from colouration, toxic hazard or food tainting are factors to be considered in the selection of plasticisers. Plasticisers are seldom added at concentrations exceeding 5% to plastics intended for food contact use.

Slip additives. These are, in effect, external lubricants that operate in the solid state. The most commonly used slip additives are fatty acid amides such as erucamide. These additives are used to prevent blocking in thin films of polymer, e.g. sticking together of thin film bags.

Other Stabilisers. To reduce the formation of large crystalites in polypropylene upon heating and slow cooling with consequent loss of impact strength and transparency it is common practics to incorporate in the polymer nucleating agents such as tertiary butyl benzoic acid or its salts or salts of aromatic sulphonates.

To prevent the thermal decomposition of PVC with the consequent evolution of hydrogen chloride, stabilisers such as barium, cadmium , zinc, or calcium salts of fatty acids, and organotin compounds or organophospites are used to act as acid acceptors.

End-Use Additives

The main types of end-use additives are listed below and discussed under separate headings.

Antiblock Additives
Antifungal Agents
Antioxidants
Antistatic Agents
Bactericidal Agents
Brighteners and Whiteners
Colourants
Expanding Agents
Impact Improvers

Lubricants
Plasticisers
Ultraviolet protective agents and ultraviolet degradation inhibitors

Antiblock additives. These are sometimes incorporated into the polymer after moulding as well as in the melt (see Processing Aids).

Antifungal agents. These are rarely used in food grade polymers, their used being confined to film or sheet for medical use.

Antioxidants. In addition to being used as processing aids, additional antioxidant is sometimes incorporated in the polymer after moulding. This applies to applications where relatively high temperatures are involved as in contact with hot foods, infrared ovens or in tropical areas where substantial exposure to ultraviolet radiation is likely to be encountered.

Antistatic agents. Again, this type of additive might be incorporated after moulding as an alternative to or in addition to inclusion as a processing aid.

Bactericidal agents. Although plastics are usually immune to bacterial attacks there is an exception in the case of plasticised PVC where the plasticiser is susceptible to such attack. The majority of bacteriocidal agents used in polymer formulations are quarternary ammonium compounds.

Brighteners and whiteners. This type of additive, (otherwise known as optical bleaching agents) is used to off-set the off-white or pale yellow discolouration of many types of plastics in their moulded state. Brighteners are added to enhance appearance. These substances operate by absorbing incident radiation of suitable wavelength, converting this, and emitting radiation of a higher frequency in the visible spectrum or in the ultraviolet region. The eye interprets this as a whitening or brightening effect.

When used, optical brighteners are usually derivatives of stilbene or thiophen and are incorporated in the polymer at very low concentrations, usually in the 100 parts per million region.

Colourants. There are two main ways in which colourants can be involved in the manufacture of food grade plastics. Firstly, there is the use of printing inks for decorative or labelling purposes. These inks are applied to the plastic surface which is not in contact with the foodstuff and do not therefore present a health hazard problem. Secondly, there are the types of colourant which are incorporated in the bulk of the plastic, usually at some stage when the plastic is molten. In this method of colouring the colourant may be present in the form of a fine insoluble dispersion of pigment which, hopefully, is well dispersed or as a solid solution, i.e. a dyestuff. Most pigments are inorganic and include such substances as titanium dioxide (whitening) in the concentration range 0.01 to 1%, cadium sulphides or sulphoselenides (yellow, red, brown) at the 0.1% level and carbon black's at the 0.2 to 2% level. In addition, high molecular weight organo-metallic pigments are occasionally used in food grade plastics such as the anthraquinones (blue, green) and other stable organic pigments. Dyestuffs are usually completely organic and include many of the substances used in textile printing. These are usually incorporated in plastics in the 10 to 1000 parts per million range.

Expanding agents (blowing agents, foaming agents). These are used principally in the manufacture of expanded polystyrene foam which is used extensively in the manufacture of vending cups. These are three principal types of expanding agents in use in polymer manufacture, all of which leave residues in the manufactures polymer.

C_4 to C_7 aliphatic hydrocarbons are dissolved into polystyrene granules which are then treated with steam to expand the granules into a cellular form up to 0.5% residual hydrocarbon can remain in the expanded polymer for a period of several months.

Mixtures of sodium carbonate or bicarbonate and citric acid, blended into the polymer upon heating decompose to produce carbon dioxide to expand the polymer and leave residues of sodium citrate in the polymer.

Labile nitrogen compounds, such as azo-dicarbonamide, upon heating, liberate nitrogen to produce a cellular structure and leaving possible traces of the decomposed azo compound in the polymer.

Impact improvers. These additives are used to overcome the inherent brittleness of polymers such as polystyrene, polypropylene, and terylene. The additives are incorporated in the polymer during manufacture. Pigments, extenders, fillers, nucleating agents, hydrocarbon oils, waxes and rubbers are all used as a means of improving the impact strength of these polymers.

Lubricants. External lubricants are used to reduce adhesion between stacks of moulded articles or to reduce friction between moving parts. Calcium stearate at the 0.05 to 1.0% level, and extenders and plasticisers and occasionally antistatic agents all have external lubricating properties.

Plasticisers. Plasticisers are incorporated into the more rigid plastics, particularly PVC, to make them more flexible. The types of compounds used as plasticisers also act as impact improvers due to their ability to reduce polymer brittleness. Plasticised PVC pipe is used extensively for transferring beer from the keg to the dispenser. Plasticisers are also used to some extent in cellulose acetate and polyethylene terephthalate, in film, sheet and pipe form.

Ultraviolet protective agents. Ultraviolet protective agents are used either to protect the plastic itself from strong sources of ultraviolet light such as sunlight and also to protect the packaged foodstuff from such radiation and possibly from the effects of strong lighting when on display in supermarkets.

An instance where such protection is required is in the packaging of Vitamin C containing cordials where, without protection, ultraviolet light would produce severe degradation of the vitamin.

Ultraviolet protective agents fall into two categories, those operating as uv screens, and those which operate by interfering with a degradation chain reaction in the polymer that has been initiated or catalysed by the radiation.

Ultraviolet screens. Ultraviolet screens act by absorbing or reflecting harmful radiation and converting it to harmless radiation of a different wavelength. All opaque, non-highly coloured additives such as fillers, and carbon black have a beneficial effect as ultraviolet screens when incorporated at the 2 to 3% level. Such compounds protect not only the plastic package from ultraviolet degradation but also the packaged food itself, and in fact, over 90% of all radiation transmission can be eliminated by the incorporation of 0.1 to 0.2% of particular pigments notably carbon black.

Ultraviolet degradation inhibitors. This is another category of materials to the filler and pigment screens mentioned above. These materials are generally organic and include derivitives of thiophen, benztriazole and transition metal

dithiocarbamates (e.g. Ferro 101, Nickel dithiocarbamate). These substances are
effective at concentrations of 0.1% or less.

Chapter 3

Principles of Extractability Testing
of Plastics

The extractability of an additive from a plastic can be determined by contacting the plastic for a specified time and temperature with either the foodstuff or beverage itself or with a range of oily, alcoholic and aqueous extractants which simulate various types of foods. At the end of the extraction test the liquids are analysed for the extracted additive by an appropriate analytical technique.

The determination of additives and their breakdown products and of other polymer impurities (e.g. monomers) in foods and food simulating extractants obtained in polymer extraction tests presents many difficulties to the analyst. Thus, it may be necessary to devise methods for determining these substances in amounts down to a few parts per million in a range of aqueous and organic media. Moreover, these substances, in addition to being present in only small concentrations may be accompanied by other substances extracted from the polymer, whose presence complicates the analytical procedure and necessitates a preliminary separation before the final analyses can be performed.

Sometimes, during polymer processing an additive breaks down to some extent and, in connection with toxicological studies, it may be necessary to devise methods for determining a polymer additive in both its undegraded and its degraded forms.

All these factors can complicate the problem of extractant analysis and considerable ingenuity has sometimes to be exercised in the selection of appropriate analytical techniques. In this chapter factors governing the selection of such analytical techniques are discussed and illustrated by examples of extractant analysis.

The need to evaluate the migration of additives and adventicious impurities from plastics into food and beverages is well recognised by both raw material manufacturers, fabricators, the food packaging industry and Public Health Authorities throughout the world (see Chapter 7). There have been various approaches toward regulating the problem, both from the side of Government and from the side of industrial associations. In all cases it is fairly generally recognised that the actual hazard arising to the consumer from any ingredient of a plastic material in contact with foodstuffs is a function of two properties, namely, the intrinsic toxicity of the particular ingredient as determined by animal feeding trials, the measurement of which will not be discussed here, and the measurement of the extent to which the impurities extract from the polymer into foodstuffs or liquids simulating foodstuffs under service conditions.

Such extractability data is important as obviously an ingredient of a plastics material which is not extracted by a foodstuff with which it is in contact does not constitute any toxic hazard to the consumer.

It is well known that, apart from high polymers, plastics materials also contain low molecular compounds, particularly additives such as heat and light stabilizers, antioxidants, ultraviolet absorbers, lubricants and plasticizers. The addition of such substances is essential for processing and for achieving the desired chemical and mechanical properties.

However, low-molecular additives frequently possess a high mobility in plastics materials and, in contrast to macromolecules, are capable of migrating from the packaging material into the packed product. The use of such substances in food packaging is, therefore, subject to strong legal controls. In order to decide whether a plastics packaging material complies with the requirements of the food law, two sets of questions should be considered. Concerning the plastics materials, one must ask whether the type to be used in contact with food is approved for packaging foodstuffs and whether it contains only approved additives in the allowed concentrations. The system, plastics plus foodstuffs to be packed, must also be considered, particularly the extent to which the individual plastics additives or their secondary products and plastics monomers migrate from the packaging material into the food and the extent to which low molecular polymer components similarly migrate.

The questions concerning the plastics can in most cases be answered by the manufacturer of the materials. For selecting some packaging materials, it is more important to answer the questions regarding the system, plastics plus foodstuff to be packed. The toxicity of plastics packages, particularly those kept in contact with food for a prolonged period or heated during the pasteurization, sterilization or preparation of the foodstuff is first of all determined by the extent to which the additives migrate into the packed foodstuff. It would be ideal if the migration of each additive into the packed material could be determined when the package has been filled and stored under normal conditions of use. This would ensure that no physiologically objectionable plastics material would be admitted and, on the other hand, that no suitable plastics material would be rejected because of a hypercritical assessment. However, quantitative determination of the migrated additives in the heterogeneous foodstuff is extremely difficult. Therefore, natural migration must be simulated in model tests to determine the migrated or extracted additives in food simulants which can more easily be analysed. In this connection, the term 'migration' covers the transition of additives under storage conditions (e.g. at and below $20^{\circ}C$ and 65% relative humidity) from packaging materials into packed foodstuffs or their simulants, while 'extraction' is the elimination of additives from a packaging materials under extreme experimental conditions (e.g. at $65^{\circ}C$ or at boiling heat) frequently with low-boiling liquids.

The development of suitable analytical procedures involves the use of a wide variety of physical and chemical analytical techniques and requires considerable innovation in arriving at suitably sensitive and specific methods of analysis. The development of such methods is discussed under separate headings in this chapter.

Both of the classes of substances mentioned above (i.e. additives and impurities) must be considered in polymer extractability investigations and the higher the concentration of these substances present in the polymer then the more of them is likely to extract from the polymer in an extraction test. Obviously, it is advantageous from the point of view of the polymer manufacturer to aim at producing grades of materials intended for food packaging applications with the lowest possible content of contaminants such as unreacted monomer. Efficient control of the manufacturing process will often forestall subsequent difficulties in obtaining acceptance of polymers in food and beverage packaging applications. For this reason it is also desirable to have available methods for determining the concentration of these impurities in polymers so that the amount of impurity left in the final polymer can be controlled to a suitably low level which is known to produce an acceptable material from the point of view of extractability.

The specified conditions on the plastic extraction test and food simulating extraction solvents prescribed in the test by various authorities differ considerably, as an example of the type of test procedure recommended, those of the British Plastics Federation in their second toxicity report, and of the Food and Drug Administration of the U.S.A. are discussed below in some detail as examples of procedures which receive recognition in countries other than the country of origin.

The situation regarding extractability testing in other countries is discussed in Chapter 9.

The Food simulating extraction liquids recommended by the British Plastics Federation (BPF) and the Food and Drug Administration (FDA) in their extraction tests are listed below:-

Extraction liquids recommended by British Plastics Federation	Extraction liquids recommended by Food and Drug Administration
Distilled water	Distilled water
1:1 ethanol/water	Heptane
Sodium carbonate : 5% aqueous	Ethanol : 8% aqueous and 50% aqueous
Citric acid : 5% aqueous	Sodium chloride : 3% aqueous
Olive oil containing 2% oleic acid (or liquid paraffin if analysis proves difficult in olive oil).	Sucrose : 20% aqueous
	Sodium hydrogen carbonate 3%,
	Acetic acid 3%
	A food oil e.g. a vegetable oil or (and oil)

Practical details of the procedures for carrying out the B P F and the F D A polymer extraction tests are described below. It must be pointed out, however, that there exist many variants of these test procedures which it is not proposed to go into in detail in this book.

Polymer constituents present in the extraction liquid are often presnet at very low concentrations, and analytical methods must be so devised so as to enable analysis to be carried at these levels. Some idea regarding the concentration levels of extracted polymer constituents which it is necessary to determine in extraction liquids can be obtained by consideration of the British Plastics Federation equation for 'Toxicity Quotient' (Q).

This is :

$$Q = \frac{E \times 1000}{T} \text{ or } E = \frac{Q \times T}{1,000}$$

where (under B P F test conditions for plastics sections which are greater than 0.020 inches thick).

E = g. additive extracted per 4000 sq. cm. of plastic surface.

T = 'Toxicity factor' derived from toxicological studies. Values of T vary from 0 up to 1000 with decreasing intrinsic toxicity of polymer constituent.

The B P F state that for a polymer to be considered safe for use in polymer formulations the summation of the values of Q for the various extractable components shall not exceed 10.

In the B P F extractability test each sq. cm. of polymer surface is contacted with 1 cc. of extraction liquid, i.e. E gm. polymer constituent is present in 4000 cc. extraction liquid. Thus ppm polymer constituent (P) in the extraction liquid is given by:

$$P = \frac{E \times 10^6}{4 \times 10^3} = \frac{Q \times T \times 10^6}{10^3 \times 10^3 \times 4} = \frac{Q \times T}{4}$$

Some concentrations of polymer constituent (P ppm) found in the extraction liquid using typical values of 'Toxicity Quotient' (Q) and 'Toxicity Factor' (T) are shown in Table 1 and these figures illustrate the wide range of concentration of polymer constituents that might be necessary to analyse for in extraction liquids, i.e. from 1 ppm or less, up to several thousand ppm.

TABLE 1

Sensitivity Limits required in the Analysis of Extractants

Toxicity quotient (Q)	Q = 3		Q = 10	
Toxicity Factor (T)	T = 2 (high toxicity)	T = 1000 (low toxicity)	T = 2 (high toxicity)	T = 1000 (low toxicity)
ppm polymer constituents in extraction liquid	1.5	750	5	2500

$$P = \frac{Q}{4} T$$

If a polystyrene contained the following volatiles and during the extraction test, these completely migrated into the extraction liquid then the total Toxicity Quotient (Q) for the polystyrene volatiles can be summarised as follows:-

	Concentration of component in polystyrene, % wt./wt.	Extractability, e.g. component extracted per 100 ml. polymer*	Toxicity Factor (T)
Styrene	0.4	0.4	250**
Cumene	0.4	0.4	250***
Ethyl benzene	0.2	0.2	250***
Toluene	0.05	0.05	250***
Toluene o/m/p xylenes	0.005	0.005	250***
Benzene	0.005	0.005	1***

* assuming that polymer has a density of unity and that the additives completely migrate from the polymer during the extraction test.

** taken from BPF Second Toxicity Report[1]

*** assumed values.

If $Q = \Sigma \dfrac{E \times 1000}{T}$

Then:

Q (for the polystyrene components excluding benzene) = 4.2

Q (for the 0.005% (50 ppm) benzene)   = 5.0

Q (for total migrated polymer components)   = 9.2

This data shows that based on the above assumption regarding toxicity factors, 50 to 100 ppm extractable benzene in the polymer would render the polymer unacceptable for food packaging applications (i.e. Q > 10). This is of interest as certainly, up to a few years ago, small concentrations of benzene were detectable in certain grades of polystyrene. However, from the point of view of toxicity, considerably higher concentrations of extractable aromatics other than benzene can be tolerated in the polymer. Usually, however, in the case of food or beverage packaging grades of polystyrene it is necessary to reduce the level of all aromatics to a very low level indeed as, in addition to toxicity considerations, tainting by migrated polymer volatiles is an additional factor governing the acceptability of the polymer as a food or beverage packing material.

THE BRITISH PLASTICS FEDERATION EXTRACTABILITY TEST PROCEDURE

Scope

1. The British Plastics Federation (BPF) has described procedures for carrying out extractability tests on plastic materials in order to evaluate the toxicity hazard of additives.

   This procedure is suitable for determining the extractability from plastic sheet of various possibly toxic substances, (e.g. monomers, antioxidants and other types of polymer additives).

   The choice of conditions for carrying out the extractability test is governed by considerations explained in Note 1.

Summary

2. The plastic sample is contacted with the five standard BPF extraction liquids for a suitable period of time and at a controlled temperature. (Note 1). Blank extraction tubes in which the polymer is not included are run in parallel.

   At the end of the test the plastic test pieces are removed from the extraction liquids.

   The concentration of polymer additives etc., which has extracted from the plastic sample into the extraction liquid is then determined by a suitable analytical procedure.

Apparatus

3. (a) Extraction tubes glass tubes 1.5 in. internal diameter with B40 cone. Length of tube to base of B40 cone: 9.25 in. Lugs on tube and stopper and spring clips.

   (b) Oil bath temperature control $\pm 2^{\circ}$C. Aluminium tray on top of bath with holes to hold extraction tubes.

   (c) Miscellaneous glassware, measuring cyclinders, pipettes, beakers.

Reagents

BPF extraction liquids

(a) distilled water

(b) Aqueous sodium carbonate 5% wt./v. made from 'ANALAR' solid Na_2CO_3 anhydrous.

(c) Aqueous citric acid 5% wt./v. made from 'ANALAR' solid monohydrate.

(d) Aqueous solution of ethanol 50% wt./v. made using redistilled ethanol.

(e) Olive oil B.P.C. to which 2% wt./v. of oleic acid has been added, except in instances where the subsequent chemical analysis for extracted polymer additives is impracticable, when the analytical method may specify the use of medicinal liquid paraffin B.P. Lev. in the place of olive oil.

Procedure

5. (a) Carry out each extractability test and blank run in duplicate. Into
       five extraction tubes measure 200 ml. of each of the following extractants
       (i.e. prepare twenty tubes). Ten of these will be used for plastic
       extraction tests and the other ten will serve as blank solutions:

         i) Distilled water

        ii) 50% aqueous ethanol

       iii) 5% sodium carbonate

        iv) 5% citric acid

         v) Olive oil containing 2% oleic acid or liquid paraffin.

       Plastics samples must be handled at all times using clean thin rubber
       gloves (to avoid grease contamination of the test specimens).

   (b) If the sample is in the form of a sheet or a formed article of thickness
       greater than 0.020 inch (see Note 1), then in the sample extraction
       tubes place an amount of the sample having a surface area of 200 sq.cm.
       (both sides of specimen included in calculation of surface area, unless
       the sample is a laminate in which only one side is made of plastic).
       If the sample is in the form of a cup of a moulded article, then cut into
       pieces so that they fit into the extraction tube. Ensure that the
       extraction liquid can circulate freely between the test pieces in the
       tube. Pieces of plastic can conveniently be separated from each other
       by means of short lengths of 1mm. thick glass rod. Insert B40 stoppers
       in all twenty extraction tubes and attach springs across the lugs on the
       tube and stopper.

   (c) If the sample is in the form of a film less than 0.020 inch thick then
       pack as much sample into the tube as it will conveniently contain, (Note 1).
       In the case of each of the five B.P.F. extraction liquids place a suitable
       amount of film into the extraction tubes and retain blank tubes containing
       only the extraction liquid (no polymer). Insert B40 stoppers in all
       twenty extraction tubes and attach springs across the lugs on the tube and
       stopper.

   (d) The time and temperature of heating of the extraction tubes is chosen
       according to the type of foodstuff application intended for the plastic
       under test. The British Plastics Federation recommends various test
       schedules depending on the plastic application envisaged (Note 1).

   (e) Insert the extraction tubes in an oil bath or water bath maintained at
       the selected temperature and leave for the appropriate time. Occasionally,
       remove the tubes from the bath, wipe clean with a cloth, and invert
       several times to mix the contents. At the end of the test remove the
       tubes from the bath and wipe clean. Whilst the tubes are still warm
       remove the polymer from them using a suitable pair of clean tongs.

   (f) As soon as possible after the completion of the extraction test analyse
       the five polymer extraction liquids and the corresponding extraction
       blank solutions for the required additives by a sensitive analytical
       procedure.

Calculations

Express the results of the extraction test as follows:-

(a) For thin section plastic test specimens, (i.e. specimens which are up to and including 0.020 in. thick).

The weight in grams (E) of compound extracted from 100 cc. of plastic sample.

(b) For thick section plastic test specimens (i.e. specimens which are above 0.020 in. thick).

The weight in grams (E) of compound extracted from 4,000 sq. cm. of surface area of plastic sample (including area of both sides of plastic sample).

Note 1 Choice of Conditions for Extraction Test

There is a wide spectrum of applications in which plastics come into contact with food. Plastics are used in the processing of food in the factory : plastic films are used as food packaging materials : bottles and moulded containers are also used for marketing food and food essences. Plastic containers are used for storing food in the home, often for long periods. There are plastic mixing bowls and tableware with which food comes into contact for a relatively much shorter time, but where hot food stuffs may be involved. There are plastic trays and tablecloths, and plastic sheets covering the working surfaces of tables and benches in kitchens and cafeterias. For all these applications where food may come into direct contact with the plastics material some standard is necessary. It is not practicable to adopt a single set of conditions under which to test all plastics, since account must be taken of the type of use to which the material will be put. For the purpose of establishing criteria of suitability from the point of view of freedom from toxic hazard, however, types of use may be divided into four broad categories as follows, and the principles of extraction tests appropriate to each are laid down:

Category A - Plastics used for food packaging and long term storage This group includes plastics for the packaging of food between manufacture and use, and for prolonged storage in the household.

Category B - Plastics intended for temporary contact with hot food This category includes domestic mixing bowls and equipment containers for short term storage and tableware.

Category C - Plastics intended for temporary contact with cold food These include trays, tablecloths, regrigerator liners and working surfaces.

Category D - Plastics for food manufacturing or processing plant Plastics in this category are used under a wide range of service conditions and it is not possible to lay down a single standard test for all these. The principles of this method can nevertheless be applied.

Note 2 Conditions of Test

Category A Plastics materials for applications in this category should be subjected to extraction tests at 60°C. for ten days. This temperature is the highest at which plastics are likely to remain in prolonged contact with food.

It also provides a measure of acceleration so that the time of ten days gives
an adequate indication of the extractability ingredients.

Category B Materials intended for applications involving temporary contact with
hot food should be subjected to extraction test at 80°C. for two hours, followed
by cooling to room temperature in the extractant and continued immersion at this
temperature for a further sixteen hours.

Category C   Plastics for applications involving temporary contact with cold
food should be subjected to extraction tests at 45°C. for twenty-four hours.

Category D Plastics for food manufacturing or processing plant should be
subjected to extraction test to be agreed between the supplier and the
purchaser under conditions of temperature and time appropriate to the individual
use of the material.

The principles of testing outlined above are in general designed to give a
measure of acceleration and/or exceptional severity. There are, however, plastics
which are well established in certain applications involving contact with food
which under test conditions undergo attack which would not be met in service.
In these conditions alone, the plastics should be tested under specific
conditions of use over a period twice as long as the expected period of contact.

Note 3 Considerations of Dimension and Shape

Experimental work has shown that the extractability of ingredients of plastics
materials is dependent upon the dimensions of the sample tested, and in
particular on the ratio of surface area to volume of the specimen. In the
case of thin materials such as wrapping films, extractant action is
substantially dependent on the thickness of the film, but in the case of
thick section materials the effect of the amount of surface area exposed to the
extractant predominates and the amount extracted is not significantly dependent
on thickness. There is of course, no sharp point of change between the two
conditions but experiment has shown that a specimen thickness of 0.020 inch
represents a reasonable division. Therefore, when testing plastics which will
be up to and including 0.020 inch thick when in contact with food the amount
extracted should be considered proportional to the volume of the sample; when
the plastics will be over 0.020 inch thick the amount extracted should be
considered proportional to the surface area of the sample.

Note 4 Methods of Test

While it will generally be possible to test the sample by complete immersion in
the extractant for the period and at the temperature required according to the
type of application for which the suitability of the production is being assessed,
plastics come into contact with foodstuffs in an infinite variety of forms and
special techniques will, in some cases, have to be adopted. For instance, in the
case of laminates of different materials it will be necessary to expose only one
side of the sample under test to the extractant. In the case of tubes in which the
inside and outside walls are different composition it will be necessary either to
fill a sample section with extractant, stopping up the ends with a material
which will have no effect on the test, or similarly to block the ends of a weighted
section of tube and immerse it in the extractant, depending upon the surface to
be tested. If the sample is in the form of a cup of beaker the test may
readily be carried out using the article itself as the container for the
extractant.

In all cases, however, the appropriate temperature and time of test as
specified above should be used, and the volume of extractant must not be less
than 1cc. per sq.cm of surface in the case of thick section (over 0.020 inch)
materials, or 20 times the volume of thin section samples. The containers of
sample and extractant should be agitated intermittently.

All extraction tests should be carried out at least in duplicate, using a fresh
sample and supply of extractant for each individual test, and the mean of the
results obtained should be taken as the amount extracted.

THE FOOD AND DRUG ADMINISTRATION (U.S.A.) EXTRACTABILITY
TEST PROCEDURE

The following procedure has been found to be of general applicability.

Scope

1. The procedure is suitable for determining the extractability from plastic
   sheet of various toxic substances, (e.g. monomers, antioxidants and other
   additives, and impurities).

Summary

2. Standard sized test pieces of the plastic under test are placed in suitable
   tubes and are contacted with the F.D.A. extraction liquids viz.:

     i) distilled water
    ii) 3% aqueous acetic acid
   iii) 3% aqueous sodium bicarbonate
    iv) 3% aqueous sodium chloride
     v) aqueous ethyl alcohol of the appropriate concentration
    vi) 20% sucrose solution containing 1% citric acid adjusted to pH 3.5
   vii) a liquid food fat e.g. vegetable oil or lard oil. Blank tests in which
        the plastic sheet is not included are also carried out.
  viii) Heptane

The tubes are heated at 135 ±5°F for seven days.

Substances extracted from the plastic into the extraction liquid are then
determined by any suitable analytical procedure capable of determining trace
amounts of these substances.

If no extractability of the determined substances from the plastic into the
extraction liquid occurs during one week then the test may be terminated.
If, however, any extractability of the determined substance does occur during
this period then the extraction test must be extended until maximum
extractability has been achieved, (at least one additional week).

Apparatus

3. **Extraction tubes** Glass tubes 1.5 in internal diameter with B40 joint.
   Length of tube to base of ground glass joint, 9.25 in.

   Oil bath Temperature control ±5°F. Aluminium tray on top of bath with holes
   to hold extraction tubes.

Reagents

4. (a) <u>Acetic acid 3%</u> dilute   30ml. glacial acid 'ANALAR' to 1 litre with distilled water.

   (b) <u>Sodium bicarbonate 3%</u> dissolve 30g. sodium bicarbonate. 'ANALAR' in distilled water and make up to 1 litre.

   (c) <u>Sodium chloride 3%</u> dissolve 30g. sodium chloride 'ANALAR' in distilled water and make up to 1 litre.

   (d) <u>Aqueous ethanol</u> Make up a solution of redistilled ethyl alcohol and distilled water of the appropriate concentration, typically 8% or 50%.

   (e) <u>Sucrose 20% - citric acid 1% solution</u> Dissolve 200g. sucrose and 2g. citric acid in distilled water and make up to 1 litre.

   (f) <u>A liquid food fat</u>, a vegetable oil or a lard oil are suitable. <u>N.B.</u> pure grade reagents are used to prepare the extraction liquids in order to minimise interference in analysis of the extraction liquids by impurities in the reagents used in the preparation.

Procedure

5. The F.D.A. extraction test states that the exposure conditions used in the test must be such that 1 sq.in. of the plastic sheet test piece is exposed to 2 ml. of extraction liquid (one side only of the test piece is used in this calculation). The specified surface area to extraction liquid volume relationship is achieved in this method by contacting ten 8 in. x 1 in. x 0.1 in strips of the plastic with 160 ml. of extraction liquid.

Some method is required of spacing these strips from each other in the extraction tube in order to permit free circulation of the extraction liquid between the test pieces during the test. This may be achieved by cutting the ten strips from a sheet of plastic having a curved edge, e.g. a plastic tile. Alternatively the strips may be separated from each other by means of 1mm diameter glass rod U clips.

Before the test the strips should be handled only wearing rubber gloves (to avoid grease contamination of the test specimen).

   (a) Pack ten 8 in. x 1in. strips in a clean dry extraction tube. Pour 160 ml. of the appropriate extraction liquid into the tube and stopper lightly, (Note 1). Run an extraction liquid blank in parallel (i.e. polymer strips absent). Immerse the sample and blank extraction tubes in an oil bath maintained at $135 \pm 5°F$. Tighten the ground glass stoppers when the tube contents have reached the oil bath temperature. Run the test for 7 days at this temperature. Occasionally remove the tubes from the oil bath, wipe clean with rag, and invert several times to mix the contents. At the end of the test wipe the tubes clean and pour the contents into a clean stoppered 250 ml. conical flask. These solutions are now ready for the determination of extractables by any suitable analytical procedure.

Note 1

<u>Preheating of extraction liquid before test</u>. If a food is to be packaged at a temperature above 135°F. (i.e. the temperature of the extraction test), the test must relatistically reflect this temperature. Thus, if the foodstuff

is to be packed in a plastic container at 160°F. then the extraction liquid must be heated to this temperature for a few minutes before pouring on to the plastic strips at the beginning of the test. The tube contents are then allowed to fall to the oil bath temperature of 135°F.

The detailed extractability test schedule published by the Food and Drug Administration is reproduced below by kind permission of this organisation.

This schedule is taken from the 121.2526 Amendment published in Federal Register January 28, 1966; 31 F.R. 1149.* subpart F - Food Additives P28.5

TABLE 2

Test Procedures with Time Temperature Conditions for Determining Amount of Extraction from the Food-Contact Surface of Uncoated or Coated Paper and Paperboard, using Solvents Simulating Types of Foods and Beverages

Condition of use	Types of food (see table 1)	Food-simulating solvents			
		Water	Heptane*	8 percent alcohol	50 percent alcohol
		Time and temperature	Time and temperature	Time and temperature	Time and temperature
A. High temperature heat-sterilized (e.g.over 212°F.)	I,IV-B,VII-B....	250°F.,2hr...			
	III,IV-A,VII-A..	250°F.,2hr...	150°F.,2hr...		
B. Boiling water sterilized	II,VII-B........	212°F.,30min..			
	III,VII-A......	212°F.,30min..	120°F.,30min..		
C. Hot filled or pasteurized above 150°F.	II,IV-B........	Fill boiling cool to 100°F			
	III,IV-A.......	Fill boiling, cool to 100°F	120°F.,15min..		
	V............		120°F.,15min..		
D. Hot filled or pasteurized below 150°F.	II,IV-B,VI-B....	150°F.,2hr....			
	III,IV-A.......	150°F.,2hr...	100°F.,30min..		
	V............		100°F.,30min..		
	VI-A.........			150°F.,2hr...	
	VI-C.........				150°F.,2hr
E. Room temperature filled and stored (no thermal treatment in the container)	I,II,IV-B,VI-B, VII-B	120°F.,24hr...			
	III,IV-A,VII-A..	120°F.,24hr.	70°F.,30min...		
	V,IX..........		70°F.,30min...		
	VI-A.........			120°F.,24hr	
	VI-C.........				120°F.,24hr
F. Refrigerated storage (no thermal treatment in the container	III,IV-A,VII-A..	70°F.,48hr...	70°F.,30min...		
	I,II,IV-B,VI-B, VII-B.	70°F.,48hr...			
	VI-A.........			70°F.,48hr	
	VI-C.........				70°F.,48hr
G. Frozen storage (no thermal treatment in the container	I,II,IV-B,VII-B	70°F.,24hr			
	III,VII-A......	70°F.,24hr...	70°F.,30min		
H. Frozen or refrigerated storage: Ready-prepared foods intended to be reheated in container at time of use:					
1. Aqueous or oil-in-water emulsion of high- or low-fat	I,II,IV-B,VII-B	212°F.,30min			
2. Aqueous, high- or low-free oil or fat	III,IV-A,VII-A	212°F.,30min	120°F.,30min		

* Heptane extractability results must be divided by a factor of five in arriving at the extractability for a food product having water-in-oil emulsion or free oil or fat. Heptane food-simulating solvent is not required in the case of wax-polymer blend coatings for corrugated paperboard containers of iced meat, iced fish and iced poultry.

Analytical Methods

Selection of extractability conditions First ascertain the type of food product (table 1, paragraph (c) of this section) that is being packed commercially in the paper or paperboard and the normal conditions of thermal treatment used in packaging the type of food involved. Using Table 2, paragraph (c) of this section, select the food-simulating solvent or solvents and the time-temperature exaggerations of the paper or paperboard use conditions. Having selected the appropriate food-simulating solvent or solvents and the time-temperature exaggeration over normal use, follow the applicable extraction procedure.

Reagents

   i) Water All water used in extraction procedures should be freshly demineralised (deionized) distilled water.

  ii) n-Heptane Reagent grade, freshly redistilled before use, using only material boiling at 208°F.

 iii) Alcohol 8 or 50 percent (by volume), prepared from undenatured 95 percent ethyl alcohol diluted with demineralized (deionized) distilled water.

  iv) Chloroform Reagent grade, freshly redistilled before use or a grade having an established consistently low blank.

Selection of test method

Paper or paperboard ready for use in packaging shall be tested by use of the extraction cell described in "Official Methods of Analysis of the Association of Official Agricultural Chemists". 10th edition, 1965, sections 7.034-7.039 under "Exposing Flexible Barrier Materials for Extraction" also described in ASTM Method F 34-63T, except that formed paper and paperboard products may be tested in the container by adapting the in-container methods described in § 121.2514(e). Formed paper and paperboard products such as containers and lids, that cannot be tested satisfactorily by any of the above methods may be tested in specially designed extraction equipment, usually consisting of clamping devices that fit the closure or container so that the food-contact surface can be tested, or if flat samples can be cut from the formed paper of paperboard products without destroying the integrity of the food-contact surface, they may be tested by adapting the following "sandwich" method:

  i) Apparatus

     (a) Thermostated (±1.0°F) water bath, variable between 70°F and 120°F. Water bath cover capable of holding at least an 800-milliliter beaker partially submersed in bath.

     (b) Analytical balance sensitive to 0.1 milligram with an approximate capacity of 100 grams.

(c) Tongs.

(d) Hood and hot-plate facilities.

(e) Forced draft oven.

For each extraction, the following additional apparatus is necessary:

(f) One No.2 paper clip.

(g) One 800-milliliter beaker with watch-glass cover.

(h) One 250-milliliter beaker.

(i) Five $2\frac{1}{2}$-inch-square aluminum screens (standard aluminum window screening is acceptable).

(j) One wire capable of supporting sample stack.

ii) <u>Procedure</u>

(a) For each extraction, accurately cut eight $2\frac{1}{2}$-inch-square samples from the formed paper or paperboard product to be tested.

(b) Carefully stack the eight $2\frac{1}{2}$-inch-square samples and the five $2\frac{1}{2}$-inch-square aluminum screens in sandwich form such that the food-contact side of each sample is always next to an aluminum screen, as follows: Screen, sample, screen, sample screen, sample etc. Clip the sandwich together carefully with a No.2 paper clip, leaving just enough space at the top to slip a wire through.

(c) Place an 800-milliliter beaker containing 100 milliliters of the appropriate food-simulating solvent into the constant temperature bath, cover with a watch glass and condition at the desired temperature.

(d) After conditioning, carefully lower the sample sandwich with tongs into the beaker.

(e) At the end of the extraction period, using the tongs, carefully lift out the sample sandwich and hang it over the beaker with the wire.

(f) After draining, pour the food-simulating solvent solution into a tared 250-milliliter beaker. Rinse the 800-milliliter beaker three times; using a total of not more than 50 milliliters of the required solvent.

(g) Determine total nonvolatile extractives in accordance with paragraph (d) 5. of this section.

<u>Selection of samples</u>

Quadruplicate samples should be tested, using for each replicate sample the number of cups, containers, or preformed or converted products nearest to an area of 100 square inches.

<u>Determination of amount of extractives</u>

i) <u>Total residues</u> At the end of the exposure period, remove the test container or test cell from the oven and combine the solvent for each replicate in a clean Pyrex (or equivalent) flask or beaker being sure to rinse the test container or cell with a small quantity of clean solvent. Evaporate the food-simulating solvents to about 100 milliliters in the flask or beaker and transfer to a clean, tared evaporating dish (platinum or Pyrex), washing the flask three times with small portions of solvent used in the extraction procedure, and evaporate to a few milliliters on a nonsparking, low-temperature hotplate. The last few milliliters should be evaporated in an oven maintained at a temperature of approximately $221^{O}F$. Cool the evaporating dish in a desiccator for 30 minutes and weigh the residue to the nearest 0.1 milligram, (e). Calculate the extractives in milligrams per square inch of the container or sheeted paper or paperboard surface.

(a) <u>Water and 8- and 50 percent alcohol</u> Milligrams extractives per square inch = $\frac{e}{3}$.

(b) <u>Heptane</u> Milligrams extractives per square inch = $\frac{e}{(s)(F)}$

where:

e   =Milligrams extractives per sample tested.

s   =Surface area tested, in square inches.

F   =Five, the ratio of the amount of extractives removed by heptane under exaggerated time-temperature test conditions compared to the amount extracted by a fat or oil under exaggerated conditions of thermal sterilisation and use.

e' =Chloroform-soluble extractives residue.

ee'=Corrected chloroform-soluble extractives residue.

e' or ee' is substituted for e in the above formulae when necessary

If when calculated by the equations in (a) and (b) of this subdivision, the extractives in milligrams per square inch exceed the limitations prescribed in paragraph (c) of this section, proceed to subdivision (ii) of this subparagraph (method for determining the amount of chloroform-soluble extractives residue).

ii) Chloroform-soluble extractives residue

Add 50 milliliters of chloroform (freshly distilled reagent grade or a grade having an established consistently low blank) to the dried and weighed residue, (e), in the evaporating dish obtained in subdivision (i) of this subparagraph. Warm carefully and filter through Whatman No.41 filter paper (or equivalent) in a Pyrex (or equivalent) funnel, collecting the filtrate in a clean, tared evaporating dish (platinum or Pyrex). Repeat the chloroform extraction, washing the filter paper with this second portion of chloroform. Add this filtrate to the original filtrate and evaporate the total down to a few milliliters on a low-temperature hotplate. The last few milliliters should be evaporated in an oven maintained at approximately $221^{O}F$. Cool the evaporating dish in a desiccator for 30 minutes and weigh to the nearest 0.1 milligram to get the chloroform-soluble extractives residue (e'). This e is substituted for e in the formulas in (a) and (b) of subdivision i) of this subparagraph. If the chloroform-soluble extractives in milligrams per square inch still exceeds the limitation prescribed in paragraph (c) of this section, proceed to subdivision iii) of this subparagraph (method for determining corrected chloroform-soluble extractives residue).

iii) <u>Corrected chloroform-soluble extractives residue</u>

(a) <u>Correction for zinc extractives</u>. Ash the residue in the evaporating dish by heating gently over a Meker-type burner to destroy organic matter and hold at red heat for about 1 minute. Cool in the air for 3 minutes and place the evaporating dish in the desiccator for 30 minutes and weigh to the nearest 0.1 milligram. Analyse this ash for zinc by standard Association of Official Agricultural Chemists methods or equivalent. Calculate the zinc in the ash as zinc oleate, and subtract from the weight of chloroform-soluble extractives residue (e') to obtain the zinc-corrected chloroform-soluble extractives residue (ee). This ee is substituted for e in the equations in (a) and (b) of subdivision i) of this subparagraph.

(b) <u>Correction for wax, petrolatum, and mineral oil</u>

(1) *Apparatus* Standard 10 millimeter inside diameter x 60 centimeter chromatographic column (or standard 50-milliliter buret with an inside diameter of 10-11 millimeters) with a stopcock of glass, perfluorocarbon resin, or equivalent material. The column (or buret) may be optionally equipped with an integral coarse, fritted glass disc and the top of the column (or buret) may be optionally fitted with a 100-milliliter solvent reservoir.

(2) *Preparation of column* Place a snug pledget of fine glass wool in the bottom of the column (or buret) if the column (or buret) is not equipped with integral coarse, fritted glass disc. Overlay the glass wool pledget (or fritted glass disc) with a 15-20 millimeter deep layer of fine sand. Measure in a graduated cylinder 15 milliliters of chromatographic grade aluminum oxide (80-200 mesh) that has been tightly settled by tapping the cylinder. Transfer the aluminum oxide to the chromatographic tube, tapping the tube during and after the transfer so as to tightly settle the aluminum oxide. Overlay the layer of aluminum oxide with a 1.0-1.5 centimeter deep layer of anhydrous sodium sulfate and on top of this place an 8-10 millimeter thick plug of fine glass wool. Next carefully add about 25 milliliters of heptane to the column with stopcock open, and allow the heptane to pass through the column until the top level of the liquid just passes into the top glass wool plug in the column and close stopcock.

(3) *Chromatographing of sample extract*

i) *For chloroform residues weighing 0.5 gram or less*. To the dried and weighed chloroform-soluble extract residue in the evaporating dish, obtained in subdivision (ii) of this subparagraph, add 20 milliliters of heptane and stir. If necessary, heat carefully to dissolve the residue. Additional heptane not to exceed a total volume of 50 milliliters may be used if necessary to complete dissolving. Cool to room temperature. (If solution becomes cloudy use the procedure in (iii)(b)(3)(ii) of this subparagraph to obtain an aliquot of heptane solution calculated to contain 0.1-0.5 gram of chloroform-soluble extract residue). Transfer the clear liquid solution to the column (or buret). Rinse the dish with 10 milliliters of additional heptane and add to the column. Allow the liquid to pass through the column into a clean, tared evaporating dish (platinum or Pyrex) at a dropwise rate of about 2 milliliters per minute until the liquid surface reaches the top glass wool plug; then close the stopcock

temporarily. Rinse the Pyrex flask which contained the filtrate
with an additional 10-15 milliliters of heptane and add to the
column. Wash (elute) the column with more heptane collecting
about 100 milliliters of total eluate including that already
collected in the evaporating dish. Evaporate the combined eluate
in the evaporating dish to dryness on a steam bath. Dry the
residue for 15 minutes in an oven maintained at a temperature of
approximately 221°F. Cool the evaporating dish in a desiccator
for 30 minutes and weigh the residue to the nearest 0.1 milligram.
Subtract the weight of the residue from the weight of chloroform-
soluble extractives residue (e') to obtain the wax-, petrolatum-
and mineral oil-corrected chloroform-soluble extractive residue
(ee'). This ee' is substituted for e in the equations in (a)
and (b) of subdivision i) of this subparagraph.

ii) *For chloroform residues weighing more than 0.5 gram* Redissolve
the dried and weighed chloroform-soluble extract residue as
described in (iii) (b) (3) (i) of this subparagraph using
proportionately larger quantities of heptane. Transfer the
heptane solution to an appropriate-sized volumetric flask (i.e.,
a 250-milliliter flask for about 215 grams of residue) and adjust
to volume with additional heptane. Pipette out an aliquot (about
50 milliliters) calculated to contain 0.1-0.5 grams of the
chloroform-soluble extract residue and analyse chromatographically
as described in (iii) (b) (3) (i) of this subparagraph. In this
case the weight of the dried residue from the heptane eluate must
be multiplied by the dilution factor to obtain the weight of wax,
petrolatum and mineral oil residue to be subtracted from the
weight of chloroform-soluble residue (e') to obtain wax-, petrolatum-
and mineral oil-corrected chloroform-soluble extractives residue
(ee'). This ee' is substituted for e in the equations in (a) and
(b) of subdivision (i) of this subparagraph. (note : In the case
of chloroform-soluble extracts which contain high melting waxes
(melting point greater than 170°F), it may be necessary to dilute the
heptane solution further so that a 50-milliliter aliquot will contain
only 0.1-0.2 gram of the chloroform-soluble extract residue).

Little work has been published on the theory governing the rate of migration of
extractable components from plastics into liquids. This is understandable in
view of the complexity of the problem. In the only outstanding contribution to
this problem found to date Garlanda and Maseoro[4,5] and Robinson and Becker[6]
have considered the migration of a constituent of a plastic material into a
solvent similar to a foodstuff from the point of view of the laws of diffusion
and have mathematically examined the way in which this migration varies with
respect to the principal parameters of the system such as time and temperature,
polymer thickness, choice of extractant liquid etc. Garlanda and Maseoro[4,5]
start off their treatment by considering the simple case of the migration of additives
from a flat sheet of plastic. For a plastic sheet which contains a substance
capable of diffusing along the x axis, perpendicular to the surface of the sheet:

$$F = -D \frac{\partial C}{\partial x} \tag{1}$$

$$\frac{\partial C}{\partial t} = D \frac{\partial^2 C}{\partial x^2} \tag{2}$$

Where:

F is the quantity of diffusing substance moved in units of time and area.

C is the concentration of diffusing substance.

t is the time.

D is the coefficient of diffusion, which is constant as C_o varies in the field of concentrations considered.

Assuming that at the start of the migration test the concentrations of additive within and at the surface of the sheet, respectively, are Co and C=0 and that the sheet is immersed in a large volume of extraction liquid, then for short time intervals or great polymer sheet thicknesses (denoted by) the quantity ΔS of diffusing substance which has moved from the surface unit of one single side of the sheet from the commencement to time (t) is expressed.by:-

$$\Delta S = \frac{2Co}{\sqrt{\pi}} \sqrt{Dt} \tag{3}$$

ΔS is therefore proportional both to C and to $\sqrt{t}$ whereas as a first approximation - it does not depend upon the sheet thickness. The initial phase of desorption can therefore be represented by a linear relationship with regard to the square root of the time, both for a thin film and a thick one, other conditions being equal, but in the case of the thin film the interval of time within which this can be verified is much shorter than for the thick film.

To generalise further - solving equations (1) and (2) - it is observed that, at time t, the local concentration within the sheet is:

$$C = \frac{4Co}{\pi} \sum_{n=o}^{\infty} \frac{1}{2n+1} \sin \frac{(2n+1)\pi x}{h} e^{-(2n+1)^2 \pi^2 h^{-2} Dt} \tag{4}$$

Where:

C_o is initial concentration of additive within sheet.

C is initial concentration of additive at surface of sheet.

h is thickness of sheet.

t is time interval.

the average concentration of additive $(\overline{C})$ in the sheet is:

$$\overline{C} = \frac{h}{t} \frac{1}{h} \int_{o}^{h} C dx = \frac{8Co}{\pi^2} \sum_{n=o}^{\infty} \frac{1}{(2n+1)^2} e^{-(2n+1)^2 \pi^2 h^{-2} Dt} \tag{5}$$

The amount of diffusing substance per unit area of film within the sheet at time t is:-

$$m_1 = \overline{C} h \tag{6}$$

Under conditions of C=O imposed on the surface of the sheet, it follows that:

$$m_o = hC_o \qquad \text{when } t = 0 \tag{7}$$

$$m_\infty = 0 \qquad \text{when } t = \infty \qquad c \tag{8}$$

From the point of view of additive migration the point of interest is the quantity of diffusing substance in relation to the unit of surface which has already left the sheet at time t, i.e.

$$M_1 = m_o - m_1 = hC_o$$

$$\left[1 - \frac{8}{\pi^2} \sum_{n=o}^{\infty} \frac{1}{(2n+1)^2} e - \frac{(2n+1)^2 \pi^2}{h^2} D_t \right] \tag{9}$$

where the second term within the square brackets is understood to be between 0 and 1.

When t = 0 and t = ∞ , equation (9) becomes

$$M_o = 0 \tag{10}$$

$$M_\infty = hC_o \tag{11}$$

M_∞ and M_1 are both directly proportional to C_o, but only M is also directly proportional to h. To simplify examination of equation 9, it is expressed in the following form:

$$\frac{M_1}{M_\infty} = \frac{M_1}{C_o h} = 1 - \frac{8}{\pi^2} \sum_{n=o}^{\infty} \frac{1}{(2n+1)^2} e - (2n+1)^2 y \tag{12}$$

where:

$$y = \frac{\pi^2 Dt}{h^2} \tag{13}$$

The function $M_1/hC_o = F(\sqrt{y})$ increases with y, at first rapidly and then it curves towards the axis $\sqrt{y}$ until it finally reaches the balance value of approximating to unity as y→∞ Fig.1.

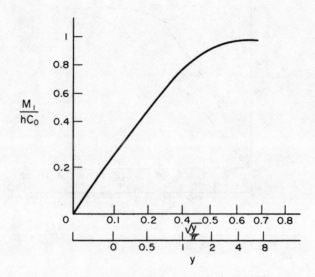

FIG.1   Reduced desorbtion graph $\frac{\sqrt{y}}{2} = \frac{1}{h} \sqrt{D \cdot t}$

For example when $\sqrt{y}/\pi = 0.8$, the value of M_1/M_∞ expressed by equation 12 is greater than 0.998, for greater thicknesses or shout periods of time corresponding to low values for y (e.g. y<1 i.e. $(Dt/h^2)^{1/2}$<0.3), $M_1/C_o h$ can be considered as an approx- imation as being directly proportional to $\sqrt{y}$, in accordance with the linear relationship with regard to $\sqrt{t}$ expressed in equation (3). By means of equation (12) and with the aid of tables and graphs it increases from y to $M_1/C_o h$ and vice- versa.

The law by which M_1/C_o and $M_1/C_o h$ vary as a function of h and t is implicit in equation 12. Garlanda and Masoero[4,5] examined this relationship explicitly in order to obtain relationships between plastic sheet thickness (h) and migration time (t) on the one hand and weight of additive extracted per unit area of sheet surface (M_1) and weight of additive extracted per unit volume of polymer (M_1/h) and weight of additive extracted per unit weight of plastic sheet, on the other hand. They examined a hypothetical situation where the coefficient of diffusion (D) equals $10^{-12} cm^2 sec^{-1}$, using three different thicknesses (10, 50, 100μ) of the same film. From equation (12) they calculated $M_t(C_o h$ and M_1/C_o, and express them in units of measure, (cm, grs, secs). In figures 2 and 2 the behaviour with regard to time is clearly seen showing the thin film quickly reaches the limit value $M_1/C_o h = 1$, whereas the quantity M_1/C_o only follows for a short period and can be deduced from Fig.1 and equation (13), (the curve with regard to $\sqrt{t}$ of equation (3). The equilibrium value M_∞/C_o will therefore be proportional to the thickness. In cases where, instead of exposing both sides of the film to the solvent, only one single side is placed in contact with the liquid, it is expected that for low values of y (for which equation 3 is applicable), the total quantity of diffusing substance that has moved will be only half that obtained when both surfaces are in contact: when time is infinite, the total quantities extracted per unit area of exposed plastic are identical.

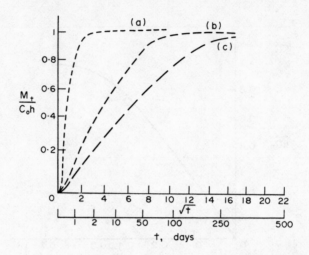

FIG.2 Diffusion as a function of time (days)

$D=10^{-10}cm^2sec^{-1}$

h=thickness of plastic sheet

a) = 0.01mm
b) = 0.05mm
c) = 0.10mm

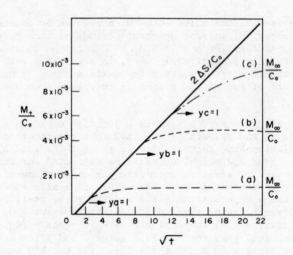

FIG.3 Diffusion as a function of time (days)

$D=10^{-12}cm^1sec^{-1}$

h=thickness of sheet

a) = 0.01mm
b) = 0.05mm
c) = 0.10mm

In Figures 4a, 4b and 4c some examples of extraction are considered with regard
to the thickness of the film or sheet. In the case of high thicknesses Mt/Coh
shows little or no sign of alteration in so far as the thickness varies: more
specifically, this happens for values of y less than 0.1, and the limit thickness
beyond which this can be verified will vary from system to system together with
the coefficient of diffusion and time (t). Furthermore, if y>2, the relationship
M_1/hCo tends to become constantly equal to 1, in as much as the extraction is
total.

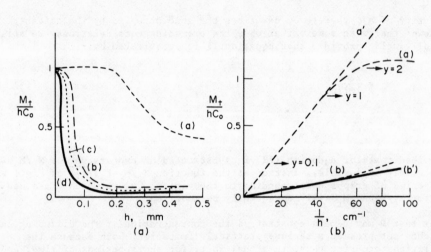

FIG.4 Diffusion as a function of thickness

a) $D = 10^{-12} cm^2 sec^{-1}$; t = 10 days from equation 12
b) $D = 10^{-12} cm^2 sec^{-1}$; t = 10 days from equation 12
c) $D = 10^{-12} cm^2 sec^{-1}$; t = 5 days from equation 12

In other words, M_t/hCo=f(h) is characterised in practice by an initial line
within which it is constant and equal to 1, a second zone of rapid descent and a
final zone of slow decrease (Fig.4a). When the same quantity is expressed as a
function of 1/h (Fig.4b), a curve is obtained which is more easily used
similar to the corresponding graph in Fig.1 where D and t are fixed.

In the same way, the function M_t/C_o=F(h) first of all increases rapidly, bends and
begins to grow much more slowly, or with the best possible approximation (3),
it remains constant in as much as for great thicknesses the system is to be
regarded as semi-infinite.

The procedure or the movement is definite if y is definite (not only h or t): in
view of the wide field within which D varies for the various systems, the values
of y corresponding to the salient zones of the functions M_t/C_q and M_t/hC$_o$ can be
achieved from very different plastic films or sheets as regards thickness and
type. This could perhaps explain the disagreement that are observed with some
systems when tests have been completed to establish how the quantity extracted
varies according to the thickness with reference to the weight of the film or
area.

Garlanda and Maseoro[4,5] went on to consider a system in which the volume of
solvent had a defined volume. To generalize, they assumed that the coefficient
of distribution (K) between the solvent and the film is not unity i.e. that the

concentration of additive at equilibrium in the solvent near the plastic sheet is K times greater than the concentration of additives in the bulk of the solvent.

Plastic sheet with a thickness of $2\ell=h$, occupies the space $-\ell<x<\ell$, while the solvent is limited to the space $-(a+\ell)\leqslant x\leqslant-\ell$ and $\ell\leqslant x\leqslant(\ell+a)$. The initial concentrations of additive will therefore be:-

$C=Co$ when $-\ell<x<\ell$ when $t=0$
$C=0$ when $-\ell(a+\ell)\leqslant x<-\ell$ and $\ell<x\leqslant(\ell+a)$ where $t=0$.

The quantity of a), therefore, describes the zone occupied by the solvent. It has been shown[7] that with some variations, the preceding considerations are still essentially valid provided that equation 11 is substituted by:-

$$M_\infty = \frac{2\ell Co}{1+1/\alpha} \tag{14}$$

where: $\alpha = \dfrac{a}{K\ell}$

and provided that for equation (12) is substituted an expression for M_t/M_∞ which is more widely employable. Instead of the function $M_t/M_\infty=F_\infty(\sqrt{y_1\pi}$ of Fig.1 we now have a series of graphs corresponding to the various values which α assumes and the values for M_t/h and M_t will consequently be modified.

The fact that D may remain constant as the concentration of the diffusing substance varies does not present a serious practical limitation, both because the concentrations occuring vary, in actual fact, for short periods of time, and because, although this would not happen, equation 2 can be generalised in this respect and the type of desorbtion resulting is still "Fickian", provided that the concentration at the surface remains constant throughout the process.

In general, diffusion in binary polymer-solvent systems is of the Fick type in the case of polymers below the transition point Tg, while deviations in the opposite direction are encountered (f). Also, in various cases when D and the concentration at the surface vary with time in a way which is known, a mathematical treatment of the phenomenon is still possible.

As a first approximation, to take account of the presence of the solvent, in the systems described above it is possible to use an apparent diffusion coefficient (D') which varies with the actual solvent used instead of the actual diffusion coefficient (D).

Especially in the case of solvents which can react strongly with the plastic material (e.g. swelling) D' can differ very greatly from the actual coefficient and give rise to behaviour which is distinctly abnormal, and as such it varies in accordance with the penetration of the solvent, and therefore changes in respect of time and position.

Garlanda and Maseoro[4,5] applied the above considerations to the practical aspects of extractability testing. Regarding the effect of extraction time (t), they state that the quantity of plastic additive that migrates varies in function of $\sqrt{t}$ and tends towards a limit value of M_∞, which is a function of the initial content of the diffusing substance in the plastic and also, in the case of equation 14, of the coefficient of distribution K. The relative graphs represent functions, which are never convex towards the axis of the abscissae.

The time required to reach M_∞ depends upon the nature of the system and in particular upon the thickness and coefficients of diffusion, and can therefore differ very widely, depending upon the particular extraction system under investigation. To prolong a test until it reaches M_∞, would involve very long extraction test times. They quote as an example the extraction of styrene monomer from polystyrene into vegetable and paraffin oils.

The quantity of styrene which migrates (mg/dm^2) is linearly proportional to $\sqrt{t}$ during the course of a 30 day test and at the end of this time only 1.3% of the monomer present in the sample had migrated into the oil. With aqueous solvents, after 10 days at 40°C the graph had already begun to curve towards the axis $\sqrt{t}$, but the percentage of monomer which had migrated remained small with respect to the total amount of monomer originally in the polymer even after a 30 days extraction test. When a solvent which was capable of reacting strongly with the polystyrene was used, e.g. heptane at 20°C, or at 40°C, the extraction was obviously rapid: even from the very first hours of testing graphs which are convex towards the axis of the abscissae are obtained, which show the great difference in performance between n-heptane and vegetable oils.

With regard to the effect of extraction test temperatures, it is concluded that the coefficient of diffusion is related to the absolute temperature (T) of a relationship which, in its simplest form, can be expressed as:-

$$D = D_o e^{-E_D/RT} \hspace{4cm} (15)$$

where R is the gas constant and E_D is the energy of diffusion. Since each system has a different E_D value, the way in which the coefficient of diffusion also varies in accordance with variations in temperature is not equal for all the systems. If, when work is carried out at a certain temperature, it is experimentally determined that a certain relationship exists between the quantities of diffusing substance which have migrated into one solvent S_1 and another solvent S_2, this relationship cannot be directly extended to tests carried out at a different temperature. This has obvious implications when it is attempted to draw conclusions from published work in which extraction test data are reported at various temperatures.

The quantity of additive diffusing from the polymer increases as the additive content of the polymer is increased(C_o).

The imposition of a legal limit for the quantity of C_o of the material liable to diffuse present in the mass is equivalent to saying that the quantity which has migrated (under certain conditions of time, temperature, contact surface and volume) should remain below certain limits. However, the total quantity of the constituent which has migrated clearly changes, not only with a change in the extraction liquid, but also with the variation in structure and composition of the plastic. It would be expected that in plastics the relationship between the quantity of additive that had migrated and the original additive content of the polymer will be effected by the presence of certain extraneous materials (plasticisers and various additives, expecially if in large quantitues), by the crystalline structure of the polymer and by all those factors which influence the bonds between chain and chain, the energy necessary to create a "hole" in the chain and the energy required for the displacement of an extraneous molecule in the mass of the polymer being variable.

The probability that the molecule of diffusing substance has of displacing itself within the polymer is proportional to the probability of its encountering a passage between chain and chain and of its then finding sufficient space for it to insert itself in the matrix of the polymer. This probability - and therefore the coefficient of diffusion - decreases with the volume of the diffusing molecule and depends upon the form of the molecule (section, length, branches, cyclic etc.)

Within certain limits the thickness of the plastic test piece effects the results obtained in extraction tests. In some cases when the thickness of the film subject to extraction is less than 0.5mm, the quantity extracted (as total residue) is dependent upon the weight of the film, whereas, with thicker test pieces extraction is proportional to the surface area. The value of 0.5mm does not constitute a clear delimitation between the two modes of behaviour but can in many cases be used as an approximate guide.

Regarding the migration of a single additive from a plastics, two processes can occur corresponding to:

for thinner
plastic sections Mt/hCo = constant (total extraction see first part of
e.g. 0.5mm   Fig.4a)

and for high
values of
polymer Mt/Co = constant (equation 3)
thickness (h)

In reality, the changeover from one of these laws operating to the other is not simply connected with the thickness of the plastic test sheet (e.g. 0.5mm) but when the following condition is met.

$$\frac{1}{h} \sqrt{Dt} = \frac{\sqrt{y}}{\pi}$$

and also will depend on extraction test time.

Garlanda and Maseoro[4,5] speculated on the possibility of deriving correction factors which would permit the calculation of what extraction test results would be obtained, for example, with a vegetable oil from the results obtained in practical extraction tests using another extractant liquid, e.g. heptane, assuming the same plastic system is considered in each case. They assumed that in both cases equation 12 is followed using apparant coefficients of diffusion (D').

The consider three different cases (Fig.6):

(a) If, for both solvents, equation 3 applies or, at all events in the straight line portion of the reduced curve of Fig.1, the relationship between the quantities which have migrated is equivalent to the relationship between the square roots of the apparent coefficients of diffusion D_1' and D_2' of the two liquids. The latter can differ from one another appreciably $\sqrt{D_1^I}/\sqrt{D_2^I}$ can in consequence be very high; in Fig.6 the hypothetical case of $\sqrt{D_1^I}/\sqrt{D_2^I} = 10$ is used to show how the factor works.

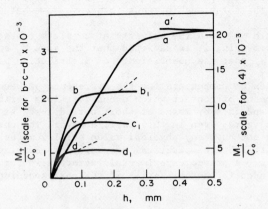

FIG.5   Diffusion as a function of thickness:

    (a) $D = 10^{-10}$ cm^2 sec^{-1}, t = 10days
    (b) $D = 10^{-12}$ cm^2 sec^{-1}, t = 11days
    (c) $D = 10^{-12}$ cm^2 sec^{-1}, t = 5days
    (d) $D = 10^{-12}$ cm^2 sec^{-1}, t = 1day

a, b^1, c^1, d^1 derived from equation 12.

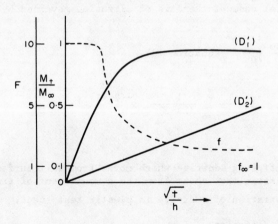

FIG.6   Relationship between quantities of migrated additive (M) and coefficient
of diffusion D:

$$\frac{\sqrt{D_1^1}}{\sqrt{D_2^1}} = 10 \quad (M_\infty)_1 = (M_\infty)_2$$

$$f = \frac{(Mt)_1}{(Mt)_2}$$

(b) In the zone between the preceeding one (a) and the zone of complete
    extraction, (c) the relationship tends to become somewhat obscure.

(c) For values of $\sqrt{t}/h$ to both the solvents at complete extraction, the factor
    is one, always providing it is admitted that the same M_∞ applies for both
    the solvents, i.e. that the coefficients of distribution are the same.

In practice, one tends to compensate for the difference between $D_1{}^1$ and $D_2{}^1$ by
simulating the phenomena of contact which occur over long periods of time in
the presence of oil and fats by means of short period tests at low temperatures
with very active solvents, even in this case, however, the observation that
this procedures does not have any physical value still remains valid, yet it
has been amply justified by the practical necessity of reducing the time and
cost of control tests. A proved experimental factor valid for one series of
tests cannot be extended to another series if the corresponding values for $\sqrt{y}$
do not coincide.

From this, it follows that only a solvent which possesses the characteristics
of the foodstuff can be selected as representative of the phenomena of
migration, and it should be used at a temperature not far removed from that
encountered in practical use. Whereas, for aqueous, acidic and alcoholic
foodstuffs, these conditions can be sufficiently closely approximated with the
solvents recommended by the various authorities for extraction tests, in the
case of fats only the use of products with physical and chemical products similar
to those of the fats in question can supply valid information.

From these considerations it can be concluded that the rate of migration of a
constituent of a plastic into a foodstuff or a foodstuff simulent solvent is
governed by a special case of the laws of diffusion governed by the following
equations:

$$\Delta s = \frac{2Co}{\sqrt{\pi}} \sqrt{Dt} \qquad \text{equation (3)}$$

$$\frac{M_1}{M_\infty} = \frac{M_1}{CoH} = 1 - \frac{8}{\pi^2} \sum_{n=o}^{\infty} \frac{1}{(2n+1)^2} \, e^{-(2n+1)^2 y}$$

where:

Δs = quantity of diffusing additive which moves from unit surface area of one
      side of the plastic test sheet from the commencement of time t.

C_o = initial concentration of additive in plastic test sheet.

D = coefficient of diffusion.

t = time

M_1 = weight of additive/unit area of sheet surface = hCo where h = plastic sheet
      thickness.

$y = \dfrac{\pi^2 Dt}{h^2}$

These equations show the dependence of the quantity of the additive which migrates
from the plastic on the parameters, plastic sheet thickness (h), extraction time
(t) initial concentration of additive in plastic sheet (Co) and coefficient of
diffusion of the additive (D).

Chapter 4

Determination of Additives in
Aqueous, Alcoholic and Simple
Hydrocarbon Extractants

This Chapter deals with the determination of various types of polymer additives
and of residual monomers in aqueous and alcoholic simulant extraction liquids
in liquid foodstuffs and beverages and in solid foods. Some discussion is also
included on the determination of simple hydrocarbon extractants such as hexane
and liquid paraffin as these extractants can often be analysed by a method
which is a simple extention of the method applied to the aqueous and alcoholic
extractants. The discussion of complex fats such as sunflower seed oil is more
complex and is reserved for Chapter 6.

4.1 Application of Ultraviolet and Fluorescence Spectroscopy

Determination of benzoic acid in British Plastics Federation simulent liquids.

Many additives can be determined in extraction liquids in amounts down to
5 parts per million by direct ultra-violet spectroscopy, e.g. phenolic
antioxidants which absorb strongly in the ultraviolet.

All of the aqueous extractants recommended by the British Plastics
Federation are optically clear in the region 250/260 to 400   millimicrons, and
hence do not interfere in the determination of additives in this optical
range. Liquid paraffin shows absorptions due to aromatic impurities below
280nm but these can be removed by percolation through silica gel. Thus,
direct ultraviolet spectroscopy has been used to determine the extractability
of benzoic acid from 0.020 in thick sheets of polypropylene. Polypropylene
containing 0.25% of the additive was contacted with the five B.P.F. extractants
for 10 days at 60°C. In the different extractants examined, the position of
the aromatic absorption peak due to benzoic acid varied between 268 and 275 nm
according to the nature of the solvent. The procedure was calibrated against
synthetic solutions of benzoic acid in the various extractants and this showed
that the method was capable of determining benzoic acid down to 3ppm using
a 1 cm sample cell. The results obtained on the thin polypropylene sheet
showed that, depending on the extractant, between 40% and 80% of the original
additive content of the film migrates into the extraction liquid during the
10 days extraction test at 60°C.

The determination of Uvitex OB illustrates an example of the application of
ultraviolet spectroscopy to the determination of additives in foodstuff
simulent extraction liquids.

Figures 7(a) and 8 respectively show an ultraviolet spectrogram and a
calibration graph which demonstrates that the optical brightener Uvitex OB
(2,5 bis (6' tert-butyl benzo oxalyl (2) - thiophen) can be estimated in
amounts down to 3ppm in these extractants by direct spectroscopy at its
absorbtion maximum occurring at 378 nm.

Table 2 gives the formulation of a polyethylene and a polystyrene used in
some Uvitex AB extractability studies. In addition to the ultraviolet
stabiliser, liquids obtained in extractability tests carried out on these
plastics would contain various other substances, some of which are ultraviolet
absorbers and which may be present in the extractant at higher concentrations
than Uvitex OB. In this case the polymer also contained Santonox R, Wingstay
T,phenolic antioxidant and styrene monomer. The presence of such ultraviolet
absorbing substances in the extractant will interfere in the determination
of Uvitex OB at 378 nm. In applying spectroscopic methods of analysis to
extractants, consideration must always be given to the possibility of interference
by any polymer additives present other than that which it is required to
determined.

Ultraviolet spectra were run on solutions of the various additives in the
region of the Uvitex OB absorption maximum (378 nm) to ascertain to what
extent these would interfere in the determination of Uvitex OB. Table 3 and
Figure 9(a) show that in the case of the polyethylene the level of Santonox
R present would not seriously interfere in the determination of Uvitex OB, i.e.
if the extractant contained twice as much Santonox R as Uvitex OB then the
reported Uvitex OB analysis would be only approximately 10% higher than
theoretical. A rather different picture emerged, however, in the case of the
polystyrene sample which contains a wider range of additives than the polyethylene
sample; these are present in the polymer at appreciably higher concentrations
than the level of Uvitex OB. In fact (Table 3), if all the additives present
migrate from the polymer at the same rate as does Uvitex OB, the latter could
not be determined in the extractant by ultratiolet spectroscopy because at 378nm
the absorption due to other polymer additives would be about thirty times
greater than that of the Uvitex OB alone.

Extraction liquids can contain a mixture of extracted substances, and one
method of applying spectroscopy in these cases is recommended by Morton and
Stubbs[8].

Application of the Morton and Stubbs procedure can be demonstrated by
considering the extractant from a polystyrene formulation containing, in
addition to Uvitex OB, Wingstay, butyl stearate and mineral oil.

Figures 9(b) to (d) are ultraviolet spectra in the 250 to 418 nm region of
synthetic solutions in the 5% sodium carbonate extractant of Uvitex OB
(53 ppm), and up to three times this concentration of the other three polymer
additives. Each of these additives would seriously interfere in the
determination of Uvitex OB by evaluation of its absorption maximum at 378 nm.
In the Morton and Stubbs approach measurements are made at not only this
maximum but also at the two Uvitex OB minima at 275 and 418 nm (Figure 9(a)).
Using suitable calibration and calculation procedures it is then possible to
calculate the corrected optical density at 378 nm due to Uvitex OB alone,
provided that in the region 275-418 nm background absorption due to any other
substances present is low, fairly linear, and not too steep.

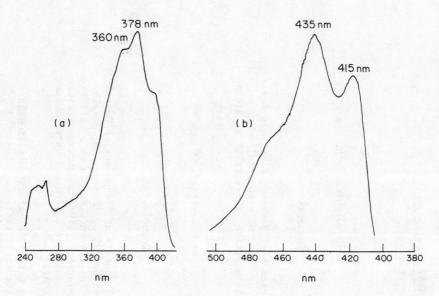

FIG.7 Ultraviolet absorption and visible fluorescence spectrograms of Uvitex OB.

(a) Ultraviolet absorption spectrum(240-400 mµ) of Uvitex OB (53ppm) in 50% of ethyl alcohol: distilled water extractant (1cm cell) showing absorption maximum at 378 nm using tungsten lamp (slit width 0.04mm)

(b) Visible fluoroescence spectrogram (380-500 mµ) of Uvitex OB (28ppm) in 50% ethyl alcohol: distilled water extractant (1cm cell) showing maxima at 415 and 435 nm using light fitter with transmission 380-540 nm and high pressure mercury vapour lamp (slit width 0.1mm).

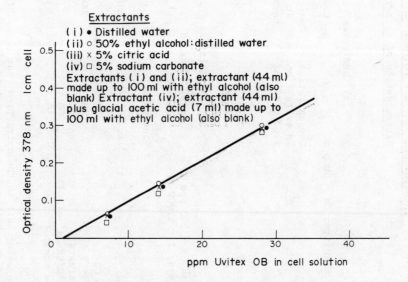

FIG.8 Calibration Curve. Ultraviolet spectroscopic determination of Uvitex OB at 378 nm in aqueous extractants (British Plastics Federation).

TABLE 3

Interference by other Polymer Additives in the Ultraviolet Spectroscopic
Determination of Uvitex OB in Foodstuff Extractants

(a) Additives present in polyethylene:

Uvitex OB - 50 ppm   Santonox R - 100 ppm   Zinc sulphide - 300 ppm

	Concentration in extraction liquid(a) ppm	Optical density at 378 nm (1 cm cell)	Comments
Uvitex OB	5	0.052	The presence of Santonex R at this level would not cause more than 10% error in the determination of Uvitex OB at 378 mμ
Santonex R	10	0.005	

(b) Additives present in polystyrene:

Uvitex OB - 200 ppm   Butyl stearate   - 30,000 ppm   Styrene monomer- 2,000 ppm
Wingstay T - 6,000 ppm   'RISELLA' oil 33 - 40,000 ppm

	Concentration in extraction liquid(b) ppm	Optical density at 378 nm (1 cm cell)	Comments
Uvitex OB	5	0.05	Optical density at 378 nm due to Uvitex OB is less than 3% of that optical density due to interference at 378 nm by all the other migrated polymer additives present. Uvitex cannot be determined under these conditions.
Wingstay T	150	00.12	
Butyl stearate	750	0.55	
Shell 'RISELLA' oil 33	1,000	1.00	
Styrene monomer	~50	~0.06	

(a) Assuming that in the extraction test 1 cm³ of plastic is contacted with 10 ml of extraction liquid and that both additives completely migrate from the plastic into the extractant.

(b) Assuming that in the extraction test 1 cm³ of plastic is contacted with 40 ml of extraction liquid and that all the additives completely migrate from the plastic into the extractant.

The ultraviolet spectra in Figures 9(b) to (d) show that, due to the presence of
the Wingstay T maximum at 275nm, the correction procedure would not be applicable
to the determination of Uvitex OB in solutions which also contain a similar level
of Wingstay T.   However, it is quite feasible to determine Uvitex OB accurately
in the presence of up to twice its concentration of butyl stearate or mineral
oil, as the background due to these substances occurring between 275 and 418nm
is low and is sufficiently linear to permit application of the correction
procedure.   Thus in some, but not all cases, this interference can be overcome
by the use of a correction procedure of the type proposed by Morton and Stubbs.

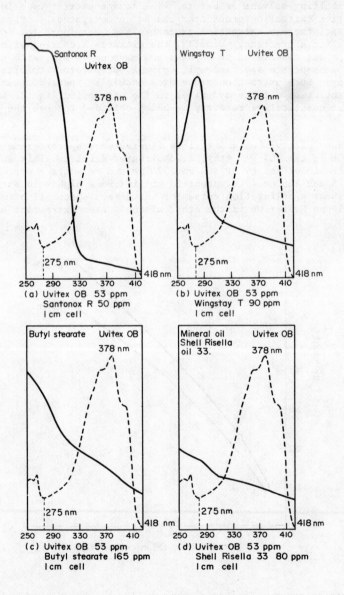

FIG.9   Ultraviolet spectrograms in the 250-418nm region of Uvitex OB and other
polystyrene additives in the 5% sodium carbonate extractant.

In the case of additives which absorb weakly in the ultraviolet, or in the case of
strongly absorbing additives which have to be determined at concentrations of
much less than 5 ppm, it is necessary to prepare a concentrate from the extraction
liquid by extracting up to one litre of it containing about 10% added sodium
chloride with a suitable low boiling solvent such as diethyl ether, hexane,
methylene dichloride or carbon disulphide. The extraction can be acheived
in about 24 hours in an upward displacement or downward displacement liquid-
liquid extractor. The 50% w/v ethyl alcohol : water extractant is distilled to
about 20% of its original volume to remove ethyl alcohol, and the residue extracted
with a low-boiling solvent as before. The hexane extract used in Food and Drug
Administration extraction procedures can be concentrated by evaporation in a water
bath. No satisfactory extraction procedure has been found for concentrating the
liquid paraffin extractant. Finally, the extracts are dried with anhydrous
sodium sulphate, evaporated to dryness and made up to 2 ml with distilled water
or another appropriate spectroscopic solvent, preparatory to ultraviolet
spectroscopy. Such extraction procedures should be checked against solutions of
known concentrations of the additives in the extraction liquids in order to
confirm that quantitative recovery is being obtained through the analytical
procedure.

Figure 7 shows ultraviolet and visible fluorescence spectrograms of a solution
of Uvitex OB in the 50% w/v ethyl alcohol:water extract. This substance
absorbs ultraviolet energy at 360 and 378 nm and re-emits a strong fluorescent
light at 415 and 435 nm (i.e. about 55 millimicrons higher in each case).
Figure 10 shows a calibration curve for the direct spectrofluorimetric determination
of up to 25 ppm Uvitex OB in the ethyl alcohol:water extractant at 415 and 435 nm.

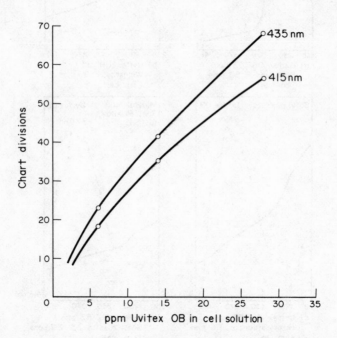

FIG.10   Calibration curve. Visible fluorimetric determination of Uvitex OB in the
50% ethyl alcohol:distilled water extractant.

In many instances, visible fluorescence methods are less subject to interference by other polymer additives present in the extractant than are ultraviolet methods. Thus, Uvitex OB has an intense ultraviolet absorption at a wavelength high enough (378 nm) to be outside the region where many interfering substances in the extractant would be excited to fluoresce. Therefore, in some instances visible fluorimetry offers a method of determining an extractant constituent without interference from other constituents when this would not be possible by ultraviolet spectroscopy. It is noteworthy that in this connection Drushel and Sommers[9] have discussed the determination of Age Rite D (polymeric trimethyl dihydroquinone) and phenyl 2-naphthylamine in polymers by fluorescence methods and Santonox R and phenyl 2-naphthylamine by phosphorescence methods. They emphasise the freedom that such techniques have from interference by other polymer additives and polymerisation catalyst residues.

Ultraviolet spectroscopy is also applicable to the determination of phenolic antioxidants in aqueous and alcoholic simulant liquids and also to one of the fatty simulants, liquid paraffin, recommended by the British Plastics Federation. Full details of the procedure, which is capable of determining down to 1-2ppm of Santonox R in the simulent liquids, is given below. With the exception of the 5% citric acid simulent, errors are generally of the order of less than ±10% of the determined concentration. Typical recoveries of Santonox R in the 5% citric acid extractant are shows below:

<table>
<tr><td colspan="2">Santonox R ppm</td></tr>
<tr><td>added</td><td>recovered</td></tr>
<tr><td>20.0</td><td>16.5</td></tr>
<tr><td>10.0</td><td>9.7</td></tr>
<tr><td>5.0</td><td>5.1</td></tr>
<tr><td>2.5</td><td>2.8</td></tr>
</table>

Method

Reagents

Citric acid AR
Ethanol AR
Sodium carbonate AR
Liquid paraffin BP (OD in 1cm cell at 280nm < 0.2 versus water)
cyclohexane - special for spectroscopy
5% w/v citric acid, prepared from citric acid AR and deionized water
50% w/v ethanol solution - prepared from ethanol and deionized water

Quartz cells of 1 cm path length are employed for all spectroscopic measurements.

Procedure

Extractant - deionized water

Shake the vessel containing the test extractant vigorously to obtain a uniform haze of "Santonox" in suspension in the water. Dispense 44.1 ml of the test extractant into a 100 ml standard flask and make up to the mark with ethanol. Wait half an hour before proceding.

Obtain spectrum of this solution and of the blank 50% w/v aqueous ethanol solution. Hence determine the optical density "d" to the "Santonox" R absorption at 250 nm.

Construct calibration curve for Santonox" R in 50% w/v ethanol in the
concentration range 2 to 20. Suitable standard solutions may be prepared by
quantitative dilution of a 100 ppm solution of "Santonox" R in neat ethanol
adjusting the ethanol content of the standard solutions to 50% w/v. (Note that
the concentration of "Santonox" R in the test extractant is 2.27 times the
concentration of "Santonox" R in the ethanolic solution prepared above.)

Extractant - 5% w/v citric acid

Shake the vessel containing the test extractant vigorously to obtain a uniform
haze of "Santonox" R in the citric acid solution. Pipette a 25 ml aliquot into
a 100 ml separatory funnel- followed by 25 ml of cyclohexane. Shake the
separatory funnel vigorously every ten minutes for half an hour.

Allow the layers in the funnel to separate. Place an aliquot of the (upper)
cyclohexane layer in the sample cell of the spectrophotometer and record a
spectrum of the extractant and of a sample of cyclohexane using a 1 cm cell
containing cyclohexane in the reference beam. Hence obtain the optical density
of the "Santonox" R absorption at 250 nm.

Construct a calibration curve for "Santonox" R in cyclohexane, by obtaining
optical densities at 250 nm of 2.5, 5, 10 and 20 ppm solutions.

Compare the optical density obtained for the test extractant with the
calibration curve and hence obtain the concentration of "Santonox" R in the
test extractant.

Extractant - 50% w/v ethanol/water

Dispense a 10 ml sample of the extractant liquid into a 1 cm quartz absorption
cell. Fill an identical cell with a sample of 50% w/v ethanol solution.

Measure the optical density at 250 nm. Calculate the "Santonox" concentration
of the solution by reference to a calibration curve for "Santonox" in 50% w/v
ethanol/water.

Extractant - 5% w/v sodium carbonate solution

Shake the vessel containing the test extractant vigorously. Obtain a suspension
of "Santonox" in 5% w/v sodium carbonate solution.

Measure 44.1 ml of the extractant and transfer to a 100 ml volumetric flask.
Slowly add 7 ml of glacial acetic acid and allow the effervescence to subside.
Dilute to the mark with ethanol.

Prepare a blank solution in a similar manner by adding glacial acetic acid and
ethanol in the above proportions to a 5% w/v sodium carbonate solution. Use
this solution in the 1 cm reference cell of the spectrophotometer and measure
the optical density of the test extractant at 250 m versus the blank in the
reference cell.

Prepare a calibration curve for "Santonox" in the glacial acid-ethanol solution
and obtain the "Santonox" concentration of the test extractant from the
calibration curve. The "Santonox" concentration of the original extractant is
obtained by multiplying this figure by 2.27.

Extractant - liquid paraffin B P

Dispense a 25 ml aliquot of the extractant into a 50 ml standard flask and
dilute to the mark with cyclohexane.

Record the spectrum of this solution prepared using 50% w/v liquid paraffin in cyclohexane in the reference cell. Hence obtain the optical density due to the "Santonox" R absorption at 250 nm.

Construct a calibration curve for "Santonox" R in 50% v/v liquid paraffin in cyclohexane for concentrations ranging from 0 to 20 ppm.

Compare the optical density obtained with the test extractant with the calibration curve and hence obtain the concentration of "Santonox" R in the test extractant. This concentration is one half the concentration of "Santonox" in the extractant.

It must be emphasized that methods based on direct spectroscopy of the extractant liquid such as that described above are only capable of giving correct analysis if no other substances which absorb at the same or a nearby wavelength are present in the extractant.

4.2 Analysis of Polymer Extractants containing more than one migrant

As discussed in Chapter 1 polymer formulations usually include one or more compounds such as antioxidants, secondary antioxidants, antistatic additives light stabilisers, lubricants, plasticizers, stabilizers, slip and antiblock agents. In addition, the polymer and hence the extractant liquid might contain other substances not deliberately added such as unreacted monomers, residual polymerisation solvents and catalysts. The result is that practical extractants from such plastics can contain very low concentrations of several very different types of substances which may or may not mutually interfere with each other during these subsequent analyses and one or more of which it may be necessary to determine.

The problem resolves itself into three stages. Firstly, the additives must be extracted from the extraction liquid in the form of an extract which is suitable for subsequent analysis. Frequently, extraction with diethyl ether or another low boiling organic solvent will achieve the required separation, certainly in the case of the aqueous and simple hydrocarbon polymer extractants In addition to isolating the additives in the form of a suitable extract, this process will achieve a useful concentration factor of up to 100 fold in the level of additives present in the extract. Secondly, it is usually necessary to separate in this extract the additive or additives which it is required to determine from those for which analysis is not required, in order to avoid any analytical interference effects. Techniques such as thin-layer or column chromatography are particularly useful in this respect and are discussed in further detail below.

Chromatographic techniques are of value in problems other than that of determining one or more additives in the presence of interfering substances. Thus, many polymer additives breakdown either during polymer processing or due to hydrolysis by aqueous extraction liquids. This facet of extractability testing is duscussed further in Chapter 7. Thus, many phenolic antioxidants are partially oxidised in the polymer during extrusion at elevated temperatures and as the toxicity of both the original antioxidant and its oxidation product may be of interest from the points of view of their extractability from the polymer and their toxicity it will be necessary to analyse for both. In a further example polymers additives such as alkyl dialkanalamides are hydrolysed by aqueous extractions to a fatty acid and an dialkanolamine immediately they migrate from the polymer.

$$RCON(CH_2CH_2OH)_2 + H_2O = RCOOH + HN(CH_2CH_2OH)_2$$

If it is required to ascertain the extent to which such hydrolysis of the additive has occured then, again, chromatographic techniques are amenable to the determination in the extractant of both the unchanged additive $(RCON(CH_2CH_2OH)_2)$ and its hydrolysis product $(RCOOH)$.

Finally, having extracted total additives from the extraction liquid and, if necessary, separating these into individual frations by chromatography it is necessary to apply appropriate analytical techniques to the determination of the individual additives.

Procedures for the solvent extraction of total polymer additives and their breakdown products from aqueous and simple hydrocarbon polymer extraction liquids and for the chromatography of these extracts are discussed below.

Preliminary Solvent Extraction of Gross Additives from

Aqueous and Alcoholic Extractants

In addition to using diethyl ether as the extraction solvent, depending on the partition coefficient of the additives between the extraction liquid and the solvent, other low boiling solvents might be suitable in certain instances, e.g. petroleum ether, methylene dichloride and benzene. The ether used for extraction can be purified by shaking 2 litres ether with 300 ml 30% aqueous sodium hydroxide in a separating funnel. The lower phase is rejected and the ether phase washed with water. Finally the ether is distilled from 20g solid sodium hydroxide and stored in an amber bottle.

<u>Extraction Test</u> (Assuming the extraction test is carried out on 700/800ml scale).

<u>Extractants : distilled water, 5% sodium carbonate and 5% citric acid.</u> Transfer the hot contents of the polymer extraction tube into a 1 litre liquid extractor (upward displacement type No. IL RDLU. Quickfit and Quartz suitable). Wash the interior of extraction tube with 25ml of hot water and ether and transfer to extractor.

<u>Extractant : 50% aqueous ethanol.</u> Transfer the contents of extraction tube to a round bottomed flask. Wash the tube with 25ml of hot water and 25ml of ether and combine. Distill until the distillate has no odour of alcohol. Make the distillation residue up to 700ml with water and transfer to liquid-liquid extractor with ether washings.

<u>Ether Extraction</u>

To the contents of the extractor (700/800ml) add 100g solid sodium chloride and stir to dissolve. Charge with ether and extract for 10-15 hours. To the ether extract add 3g anhydrous sodium sulphate. Shake, filter off the ether and wash the sodium sulphate with fresh ether into the receiving flask. Remove ether on a warm water bath, working the residue in stages into a 10ml beaker with appropriate ether washings at each stage to avoid losses of residue. Finally, quantitatively transfer the residue to a 2ml volumetric flask.

This procedure was used to check the recoveries of dilauryl thiodipropionate
(DLTDP) by ether extraction. The method was checked at the 15 and 75ppm
DLTDP level from 700ml of the aqueous and alcoholic extraction liquids.
DLTDP was determined in the extracts by infra-red spectroscopy and by
elemental analysis for sulphur (discussed later). It is seen below that
recoveries are in excess of 80%:

Extractant	Recovery
Water	80-85
Ethyl; alcohol water	90
5% sodium carbonate	85-95
5% citric acid	70-85

Separation of Individual Additives from Solvent Extract of Extractant Liquid

Some examples of the application of these techniques to the determination of
additives in extractants are discussed below.

Firstly, an example of the application of silica-gel column chromatographic
techniques to the separation of polymer additives. An extraction liquid
contained the following three additives, Santonox R (4,4' thio bis 6 tert
butyl meta cresol), Ionol CP (butylated hydroxy toluene), and dilauryl
thiodipropionate (DLTDP) and it was required to determine the concentrations
of two of them (Santonox R and Ionol CP).

Inspection of the ultraviolet spectra of synthetic cyclohexane solutions of
each of these additives (Figure 11) shows that the Santonox R could be
determined by direct ultraviolet spectroscopy with little or no interference
from either Ionol CP or DLTDP by evaulation of the maximum occurring at
250 m . However, Ionol CP could not be determined by direct spectoscopy of
the extractant by evaluation of its peak at 276nm as Santonox R also has a
maximum at this wavelength.

Interference by Santonox R in the determination of Ionol CP at 276nm was
overcome by means of a preliminary separation on a column of 100-200 mesh
silica gel (containing 4% water). To isolate total additives from the
aqueous extraction liquid it was saturated with sodium chloride and then
extracted with diethyl ether, then chloroform. The chloroform was dried with
sodium sulphate and evaporated to dryness and the residue was dissolved
in spectroscopic grade carbon tetrachloride. Percolation of this solution
down a column of silica gel gave an effluent containing Ionol CP only,
which could be determined by evaluation of its maximum occurring at 276nm.

Many useful separations of extractant constituents can be achieved by
column chromatographic techniques. Generally, however, such separations are
best achieved by thin-layer chromatography or, in the case of volatile
materials, gas chromatography, (discussed later).

Two different applications of the thin-layer chromatographic techniques
direct and indirect, are discussed below for the analysis of additive mixtures.
It is first necessary to extract total polymer additives from the extraction
liquid with a low-boiling organic solvent and concentrate the extract to
2ml as described earlier in this Chapter.

Thin-layer chromatographic plate adsorbents (e.g. silica gel, alumina etc.) usually contain small amounts of substances which migrate with the development solvent along the plate towards the solvent front. Solvents such as methanol cause migration of adsorbent impurities almost completely to the solvent front, whereas non-polar solvents such as n-hexane do so to a lesser extent. These impurities adsorbed in the ultraviolet region of the spectrum but do not appear to absorb much in the infra-red; the impurities also produce a char when the plate was sprayed with sulphuric acid and heated to about 170°C, indicating that they contain organic matter.

The presence of these impurities in the adsorbent might interfere in procedures for the quantitative analysis of mixtures carried out by thin-layer chromatography. Such interference can usually be overcome by the pre-migration procedure in which the plate is migrated to the top with methyl alcohol which removes impurities out of the region where the analysis chromatogram will be subsequently developed (a second pre-migration with methanol might be desirable sometimes to complate removal of impurities). The plate is air-dried and then conditioned in the usual way prior to carrying out the analysis procedure. Plates which have been pre-migrated are quite adequate for carrying out quantitative thin-layer chromatographic analysis of mixtures by either of the two procedures described below.

Indirect determination of Additives on the Thin-layer Plate

Suitable spray reagents which produce coloured derivatives upon reaction with separated substances on a chromatoplate are not available for all the types of substances likely to occur in extractants. If an extractant contains a mixture of additives which have to be separated, and for some or all of which spray reagents are not available, then the following approach is recommended.

To obtain sufficient material for subsequent analysis a portion of the extract of the extraction liquid (containing up to 1mg of each component) is applied in a straight line along one side of the plate by a suitable applicator. After solvent development, the bands on the plate containing each additive are marked off. The position of these bands on the chromatograph can be calculated from the known Rf values of the various sample components, as determined in a separate run carried out under identical conditions using a sulphuric acid reagent as detector. Figure 12 is a chromatoplate obtained under these conditions for a mixture of Santonox R, Ionol CP and dilaurylthiodipropionate.

The silica gel corresponding to each of these separate bands is then carefully scraped off from the plate and each transferred to a filter stick and eluted with a low-boiling polar solvent such as ethyl alcohol (Figure 13) which quantitatively desorbs the additive from the gel. Solvent is then removed from each extract, which is made up to 2ml in a volumetric flask with a suitable spectroscopic solvent. These solutions are suitable for analysis by appropriate techniques as discussed elsewhere. It is advisable to check on the recovery obtained for each additive in these procedures by carrying out suitable control experiments covering all stages of the analytical procedure on known weights of each of the additives concerned.

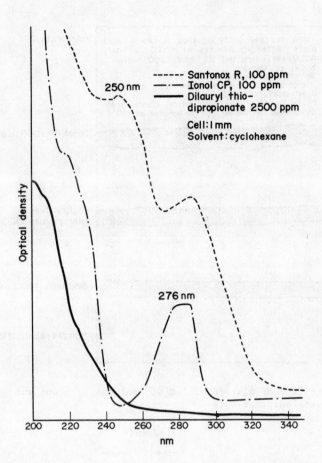

FIG.11 Ultraviolet spectra of polypropylene additives, 200-400nm.

Separation of Butylated Hydroxy Toluene antioxidant (BHT) and 2-hydroxy
4-n-octoxybenzophenone Light Stabiliser in British Plastics Federation
Extractants.

As an example of the thin-layer technique, a method is described
below for the determination of both butylated hydroxy toluene and 2-hydroxy
4-n-octoxybenzophesane in the aqueous and alcoholic foodstuff simulent
extractants of the British Plastics Federation.

The additives are first separated from the extractant liquids and thereby
concentrated by ether extraction as described earlier. As both of these
substances have similar absorption maxima respectively 280nm and 290nm in the
ultraviolet, it is first necessary to separate them and this is achieved
by thin-layer chromatography. The separated bands of additives are then
removed from the plate and determined independently by ultraviolet spectroscopy.
The overall recovery of additives through this procedure is of the order of
90-100%. It is necessary, first to work out the scaling of operations so that
the desired analytical sensitivity and accuracy is achieved.

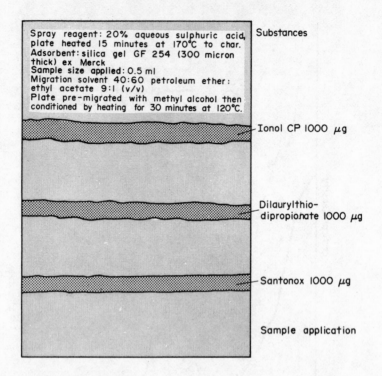

Spray reagent: 20% aqueous sulphuric acid, plate heated 15 minutes at 170°C to char.
Adsorbent: silica gel GF 254 (300 micron thick) ex Merck
Sample size applied: 0.5 ml
Migration solvent 40:60 petroleum ether: ethyl acetate 9:1 (v/v)
Plate pre-migrated with methyl alcohol then conditioned by heating for 30 minutes at 120°C.

Substances

─ Ionol CP 1000 μg

─ Dilaurylthio-dipropionate 1000 μg

─ Santonox 1000 μg

Sample application

FIG.12   Chromatoplate of mixture of 1mg of Santonox R, Ionol and dilaurylthiodipropionate

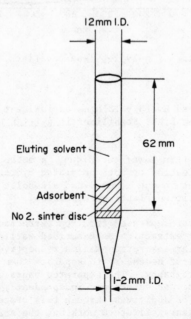

12mm I.D.

Eluting solvent

62 mm

Adsorbent

No 2. sinter disc

1-2 mm I.D.

FIG.13   Filtration apparatus for extracting separated additives from adsorbent

Scaling of operations. If it is assumed that in an extraction test 10-20g of plastics is contacted with 700ml of extraction liquid which is subsequently extracted with a low boiling solvent to remove additives and this extract is concentrated to 2ml, i.e. all the additives which migrate from the original polymer are concentrated into 2ml of solvent, then if each additive is originally present in the polymer at 0.1% then if complete additive migration occurs, the extract will contain 10-20mg of each additive per 2ml. If however, only 10% additive migration occurs, then the extract will contain 1-2mg of each additive per 2ml.

Knowing the extinction coefficients of butylated hydroxy toluene and 2-hydroxy-4-n-octoxy benzophenone it is possible to calculate the weight of each of these substances that must be present in the volume of test solution applied to the plate:

Butylated hydroxy toluene $\quad E\begin{array}{c}1\%\\1cm\\280nm\end{array} = 86.3$ (in ethanol)

Substituted benzophenone $\quad E\begin{array}{c}1\%\\1cm\\290nm\end{array} = 527$ (in ethanol)

The minimum detectable concentrations are:

$$BHT = \frac{0.1}{86.3\times3} = 386\mu g/100ml$$

i.e. 39µg in 10ml (3cm cell)

Substitute benzophenone $\dfrac{0.1}{527\times3} = 60\mu g/100ml$

i.e. 6µg in 10ml (3 cm cell)

Thus a suitable volume of the 2ml extracts for application to the plate is 0.1ml (which contains 500-1000µg of each additive if complete additive migration from the polymer has occurred and 50-100µg of each if only 10% additive migration has occurred).

The thin-layer chromatographic procedure described below for separating the additives and recovering each component for ultraviolet spectroscopy is based on the assumption that only 10% additive migration occurs from the polymer. Quantities should be adjusted if additive migration differs appreciably from 10%.

Ether extraction of extraction liquid. Discussed earlier, volume of final extract adjusted to 2ml.

Thin-layer chromatography.

Apparatus

TLC tank lined with filter paper
20 × 20cm TLC plates coated with a 0.25mm layer of silica gel GF254
Syringe to deliver up to 0.1ml
Ultraviolet lamp (wavelength 254mµ)

Sintered glass filter columns 3" × ½" with fine sinter sealed in at lower end

2ml, 10ml, 50ml and 100ml graduated flasks

Ultraviolet spectrophotometer

3cm silica cells for above

Reagents

(a) Absolute ethanol
(b) Diethyl ether
(c) Petroleum ether (100-120°): ethyl acetate mixture (9:1 vol/vol ratio)

Calibration

Prepare a calibration solution as follows:-

Accurately weigh 0.2gm BHT and 0.2gm of 2, hydroxy-4-n-octoxy benzophenone into a 100ml graduated flask and make up to the mark with diethyl ether.

Spot 0. 10, 20, 40, 60 and 80 microlitre portions of this calibration solution on to the base line of a 20 × 20cm plate in duplicate and treating these as 'sample' proceed as described under chromatography below, (Section 1). Include blanks as described.

Measure the ultraviolet absorptions of the calibration samples and blanks as described in Section 3 and calculate the nett optical density for each sample.

Plot calibration curves of nett optical density against concentration of additive in the ethanol solution used for spectroscopy for both BHT and 2-hydroxy-4-n-octoxy benzophenone.

Procedure

Preparation of standard solutions

Solution I. Weigh accurately 50mg of BHT into a 100ml graduated flask and make up to the mark with ether.

Solution II. Weigh accurately 50mg of 2-hydroxy-4-n-octoxy benzophenone into a 100ml graduated glask and make up to the mark with ether.

1 Chromatography

(a) Apply the following solutions side by side at the base line of a 20 × 20cm TLC plate in the form of a spot or short band 1 to 2cm long:-

   i) 1 × 0.1ml portion of solution I   (BHT reference)
  ii) 1 × 0.1ml portion of solution II (light stabiliser reference)
 iii) 2 × 0.1ml portions of polymer extract.

(b) Develop an ascending chromatogram to a distance of 10cm in a 9:1 petroleum ether: ethyl acetate eluent in a tank saturated with solvent vapour. Remove the plate from the tank and allow the solvent to evaporate.

2 <u>Removal of the additives from the plate</u>

(a) Inspect the plate under a 254mμ ultraviolet light source and by means of a sharp pointer mark out the dark blue zones in the two sample chromatograms which correspond in R_f to the major constituents of the two reference chromatograms.

Approximate R_f values should be as follows:-

   BHT R_f = 0.75

   2-hydroxy-4-n-octoxy-R_f = 0.60
   benzophenone

Also mark off duplicate blank areas equal in size and R_f to the spots in the sample chromatograms.

(b) Carefully scrape off the plate the areas of silica gel marked and transfer each portion of gel separately to a sintered glass filter column. Extract the additives from the silica gel with absolute ethanol and make up in graduated flasks as follows:-

   R_f - 0.75 Sample) make each up to 10ml with
   R_f - 0.75 Blank) absolute ethanol

   R_f - 0.60 Sample) make each up to 50ml with
   R_f - 0.60 Blank   absolute ethanol

3 <u>Ultraviolet Spectroscopy</u>

Measure the optical density of the duplicate sample and blank solutions at the following wavelength; butylated hydroxy toluene 280nm ,2-hydroxy-4-n-octoxy benzophenone 290nm in 3cm silica cells against absolute ethanol in the reference beam.

<u>Calculations</u>. Calculate the mean value of the sample and blank optical densities and obtain the nett optical density as follows:-

   Nett OD = (mean sample OD - mean blank OD)

Determine the concentration of each additive in the ethanol by reference to the appropriate calibration graph and relate this to the weight of additive in the extraction liquid.

<u>Direct determination of additives on the thin-layer plate</u>. Polymer additives are usually colourless compounds and cannot, therefore, be determined by comparing the intensity of colour of the separated constituents with standard control solutions of known concentration, a technique which works excellently when determining organic dyestuffs. However, many polymer additives react to produce coloured reaction products when the plate is sprayed with a suitable reagent. Comparison of the intensity of the coloured spots obtained with those obtained for the standards enables an estimate to be obtained of the concentrations of various substances present.

Figure 14, for example, shows the thin-layer plates obtained upon development of 20 microlitre of an ether solution of a mixture of Santonox R, Ionol CP and dilauryl thiodipropionate. It is seen that 2:6 dibromo-p-

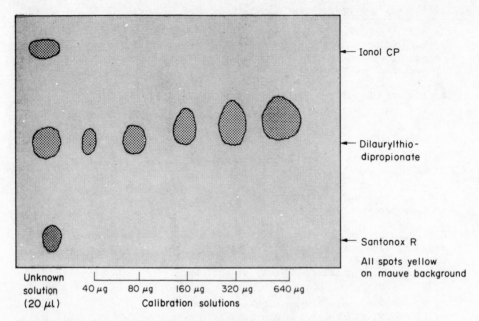

Spray reagent: Potassium permanganate (0.08 %) sodium carbonate (0.25 %)
Adsorbent: Silica gel GF 254 (300 micron thick) ex Merck
Sample size: 20 μl diethyl ether
Calibration mixtures: 40 to 640 μg of component in 20 μl diethyl ether solution
Migration solvent: 40 : 60 petroleum ether : ethyl acetate 9 : 1 (v/v)
Plate pre-migrated with methyl alcohol then conditioned by heating for 30 minutes at 120°C

FIG.14   Chromatoplate of unknown mixture of Santonox R, Ionol and
         dilaurylthiodipropionate with standard calibration mixtures.

–benzoquinone-4-chlorimine is an excellent spray reagent for showing up
Santonox R and Ionol CP but that dilaurylthiodipropionate does not show up
distinctly using this reagent; however, it produces a yellow colour when
sprayed with alkaline potassium permanganate solution (Figure 15). The
unknown and standard spots can be quantified either visually by the
bracketing technique or by densitometric scanning of the plate. These
procedures are sufficiently sensitive to detect one microgram of substances
which, with suitable scaling-up of the analytical operations, is equivalent
to determining additives at the 1 to 5ppm level in polymer extraction liquids.

Pre-migration of the adsorbent with methanol is not usually necessary when
determining additives by the direct technique. In some instances, however,
a suitable spray reagent is not available for a particular additive. In
these cases an approximate estimate of the amount of the compound present
can be obtained by spraying the plate with 20% aqueous sulphuric acid
(followed by heating at 160/200°C) and comparing the intensity of the
charred spots with that obtained for a range of standard calibration solutions
of the substance. In such instances it is, of course, necessary to pre-migrate
the plate with methanol before it is used for the analysis, to remove organic
impurities from the adsorbent layer.

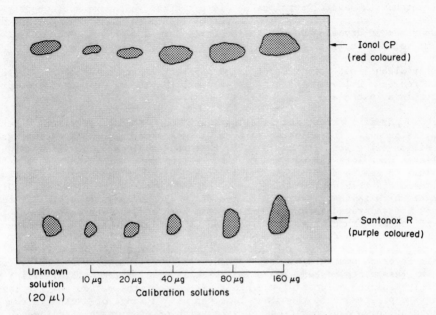

Spray reagent: Methanolic 2.6 di-bromo-p-benzoquinone-4-chlorimine, followed by
   2.0% borax solution
Adsorbent: Silica gel GF 254 (300 micron thick) ex Merck
Sample size: 20 μl diethyl ether solution
Calibration mixtures: 10 to 160 μg of component in 20 μl diethyl ether solution
Migration solvent: 40:60 petroleum ether : ethyl acetate 9:1 (v/v)
Plate pre-migrated with methyl alcohol then conditioned by heating for 30 minutes at 120°C

FIG.15   Chromatoplate of unknown mixture of Santonox R, Ionol and dilaurylthiodipropionate with standard calibration mixtures.

A procedure based on direct thin-layer chromatography, for the determination
of down to 1ppm of dilaurylthiodipropionate in the aqueous extractants of
the British Plastics Federation is described below:-

Determination of dilaurylthiodipropionate by thin-layer chromatography in
aqueous and liquid paraffin British Plastics Federation simulent liquids

Preliminary ether extraction of dilaurylthiodipropionate from the aqueous
extractants. In this method the distilled water, sodium carbonate and 5%
citric acid extractants (80ml) are transferred to a separatory funnel. In
the case of the distilled water extractant only, solid sodium chloride (10%)
is added to assist the extraction of dilaurylthiodipropionate. The addition
of sodium chloride to the distilled water extractant before ether extraction
was essential in order to obtain good recoveries. Omission of the sodium
chloride resulted in recoveries of the order of 5%. Addition of sodium
chloride to citric acid solutions was deleterious; the citric acid was
salted out in the ether, and thus remained on evaporation of the ether.
Some of this residue was dissolved along with the dilaurylthiodipropionate
and was present on the thin-layer chromatograph plate. Neutralisation of

the citric acid before extraction resulted in low recoveries. The aqueous phase is extracted with several portions of diethyl ether which are subsequently combined and dried by shaking with anhydrous sodium sulphate. The ether extract is evaporated to dryness and the residue transferred with small volumes of ether to a 2ml volumetric flask and made up to volume with ether.

The ether alcohol:water extractant is evaporated to dryness on a water bath and transferred to a 2ml volumetric flask as described above. Dilaurylthiodipropionate is determined in the ether extracts as described below.

The liquid paraffin extractant is diluted with $60^{o}C$ to $80^{o}C$ petroleum ether in a separatory funnel. The solution is then passed down a column of chromatographic grade silica gel which retains the dilaurylthiodipropionate and allows liquid paraffin to percolate through the column. Petroleum ether is then passed through the column to remove the last traces of liquid paraffin. A mixture of chloroform and methanol is then poured down the silica column to desorb dilaurylthiodip-ropionate which is quantitatively recovered in the column effluent. The total effluent is evaporated to dryness in a steam bath and the residue made up to a standard volume with diethyl ether. Dilaurylthiodipropionate is determined in the extracts described below.

The thin-layer chromatographic separation of dilaurylthiodipropionate is carried out on a glass plate coated with a 1mm thick layer of Merck No.7731 silica gel. Accurately measured volumes of the ether extracts of the various extraction liquids are pipetted onto the plate together with a range of synthetic comparison solutions of known concentrations of dilaurylthiodipropionate dissolved in diethyl ether. The chromatogram is developed with a mixture of acetone and cyclohexane (15:85 (v/v)). The plates are then sprayed with an alkaline solution of potassium permanganate, when the dilaurylthiodipropionate shows as yellow spots on a pink to red background (R_f value of dilaurylthiodipropionate = 0.65). The intensity of the sample spots is compared with that of the standard dilaurylthiodipropionate spots as soon as possible, and the dilaurylthiodipropionate content of the sample solutions deduced accordingly. It is then possible to calculate the dilaurylthiodipropionate content of the original extraction liquids.

The thin-layer chromatographic method described below is sufficiently sensitive to determine dilaurylthiodipropionate in amounts down to 1ppm in the various extraction liquids. An additional advantage of this procedure, of course, is that because it incorporates a chromatographic separation step, interference effects due to any other polymer additives present in the extraction liquid are minimised, unless these substances migrate on the plate at the same rate as dilaurylthiodipropionate itself.

Method

Reagents. All reagents should be Analar or A.R. quality wherever possible (Note 1).

Acetone
Diethyl ether
Dilaurylthiodipropionate
Cyclohexane
Potassium permanganate
Silica gel   Thin-layer chromatographic grade –
                                        Particle size 5-20 with calcium sulphate
                                        binder, e.g. Merck No.7731 (for thin-
                                        layer chromatography).

Sodium chloride	
Sodium sulphate	Anhydrous
Sodium carbonate	Anhydrous
Chloroform	
Methanol	
Petroleum spirit	Boiling range 60-80°C
Silica gel	Chromatographic grade - Particle size 0.05 to 0.20mm, e.g. Merck No 7734 (for column chromatography of liquid paraffin extractant).
Cyclohexane - acetone solvent mixture	Mix 15ml of acetone with 85ml of cyclohexane.
Potassium permanganate spray reagent	Dissolve 0.08g of potassium permanganate and 0.25g of anhydrous sodium carbonate in 100ml of distilled water. This solution is stable for only about three days and should therefore be prepared as required.
Chloroform - methanol solvent mixture	Mix 10ml methanol with 90ml chloroform.
Standard dilauryl-thiodipropionate solution	Dilute 0.1000g of dilaurylthiodipropionate to exactly 100ml with diethyl ether in a graduated flask. This solution contains 1mg/ml of dilaurylthiodipropionate.

The use of Analytical Reagent grade solvents throughout is essential to avoid streaking at the thin-layer chromatographic stage of the analysis.

Samples of dilaurylthiodipropionate in the various extractants were prepared by diluting a known volume of a stock solution of dilaurylthiodipropionate in ethanol, containing 1mg dilaurylthiodipropionate/ml to 1 litre, with the appropriate extractant. With distilled water, ethanol-water, and 5% sodium carbonate solution, satisfactory solutions were produced with 5ml of stock solution. With 5% citric acid solution, 5ml of stock solution gave a cloudy solution indicating that dilaurylthiodipropionate was not soluble to the extent of 5mg/ml in 5% citric acid. 4ml of stock solution however, gave a clear solution.

Apparatus

Thin-layer spreading device
Thin-layer chromatography plates
Thin-layer chromatography tank
Spray bottle
2ml graduated flasks
100ml separating funnels

Sampling

Aqueous and 50% ethyl alcohol and aqueous extractants. 80ml of sample is sufficient for one determination.
Liquid paraffin extractant. 70g of sample is sufficient for one determination.

Procedure

Blank Tests. These are unnecessary since the materials from which the extractant solutions are prepared are unlikely to contain dilaurylthiodipropionate.

Thin-layer chromatographic plates.

To prepare five plates, each 20cm × 20cm, shake 98g of Kieselgel G (Merck No. 7731) with 165ml of distilled water for about 90 seconds until a creamy slurry of even consistency is obtained. Pour the slurry into the spreading device and coat the plates 1mm thick without delay. Allow to stand for a few minutes until the layer has set, then transfer to an oven at 105-110°C for 60-90 minutes. Store the activited plates in a desiccated chamber until required.

Recovery of dilaurylthiodipropionate from the extractant samples

(a) <u>Extractant - distilled water</u>. Transfer 80ml of extractant solution to a 100ml separating funnel and add 8g of sodium chloride. Extract with 5 × 20ml portions of diethyl ether, combine the extracts and dry with anhydrous sodium sulphate. Decant off the ether portion-wise into a 50ml beaker and evaporate the whole of the ether in this way to dryness on a steam bath. Wash the sodium sulphate with several portions of ether transfer the washings to the 50ml beaker and again evaporate to dryness. Transfer the residue with small portions of ether to a 2ml graduated flask and finally dilute to volume with ether.

It is essential that the solutions should be applied to the plate slowly, so that the solvent spreads as little as possible. A gentle current of air blowing on the spot helps in this respect.

(b) <u>Extractants - 5% w/v sodium carbonate solution and 5% w/v citric acid solution.</u>

Transfer 80ml of extractant solution to a 100ml separating funnel and extract with 5 × 20ml portions of diethyl ether. Combine the extracts and continue as described for distilled water.

(c) <u>Extractants - 50% w/v ethyl alcohol in water</u>. Evaporate 80ml of solution to dryness, portion-wise, in a 100ml beaker on a steam bath. Transfer the residue with minute portions of ether to a 2ml graduated flask and finally dilute to volume with ether.

(d) <u>Extractant - Medicinal paraffin B P Levis</u>. Weigh 40g of sample into a 100ml separating funnel and dilute with 60-80°C petroleum spirit to approximately 100ml. Pass this solution down a column, 1cm × 3.5cm of chromatographic grade silica gel which has been activated by heating at 140°C for 1 hour.

Maintain a flow rate of 2-3ml per minute by application of gentle suction. Follow with 50ml of 60-80°C petroleum spirit, then allow the column to suck dry.

Pass down the column, at the same flow rate, 30ml of chloroform/methanol solvent mixture, followed by 20ml of chloroform, collecting in a 100ml beaker. Evaporate just to dryness on a steam bath. Transfer the residue with minute portions of diethyl ether to a 2ml graduated flask and finally dilute to volume with ether.

Thin-layer chromatographic separation

Extractants - (a), (b) and (c). For the range 1 to 5ppm of dilauryl-thiodipropionate in the sample apply aliquots of 50µl of sample solution in a line 1.5cm from the bottom of a prepared plate. In addition apply spots of 2, 4, 6, 8 and 10µl (2, 4, 6, 8, 10µg) of standard dilaurylthiodipropionate solution. For the range 5 to 25ppm of dilaurylthiodipropionate in the sample apply aliquots of 10μl of sample solution.

Extractant – (d). For the range 1 to 5ppm dilaurylthiodipropionate in the sample apply aliquots of 100μl of sample solution and spots of 2, 4, 6, 8, and 10μl of standard dilaurylthiodipropionate solution in the described manner. For the range 5 to 25ppm dilaurylthiodipropionate in the sample apply aliquots of 20μl of sample solution.

Having applied the sample spots stand the plate without further delay in a suitable tank starting line downwards, such that the lower edge dips into the solvent misture. Allow the solvent to flow 14cm to the score line, them remove the plate from the tank and allow the solvent to evaporate. Spray the plate lightly and evenly with alkaline potassium permanganate when the dilaurylthiodipropionate traces appear as yellow spots on a pink to red background. The Rf of dilaurylthiodipropionate is approximately 0.65. Compare the samples and standard spots without delay.

The spot sizes can be compared to an accuracy of ±1.0μg, representing± 0.5ppm in the 1 to 5ppm range.

The lower limit of detection of dilaurylthiodipropionate on a thin-layer chromatographic plate is 2μg, it therefore follows that it is not possible to determine the dilaurylthiodipropionate content of samples containing less than 1ppm dilaurylthiodipropionate by this method.

This procedure when applied to synthetic solutions of up to 5ppm dilauryl-thiodipropionate in the various B P F extractants gave recoveries of 80% to 100% dilaurylthiodipropionate in the extraction liquid, (Table 4).

TABLE 4

Recovery of dilaurylthiodipropionate from the various
B.P.F. extractants by the ether extraction/
Thin-layer chromatographic procedure

Extractant	dilaurylthiodipropionate content of extraction liquid, ppm	
	Added	Found
Distilled water	5.0	4.0
50% ethyl alcohol:water	5.0	4.0-4.5
5% sodium carbonate	5.0	4.0-4.5
5% citric acid	4.0	3.0-4.0
Liquid paraffin	1.0	1.0
	2.5	2.0
	3.75	3.5
	5.0	4.5-5.0

Uhde et al[10] have described a direct thin-layer chromatographic procedure for
the determination of the extractability of ultraviolet stabilisers from plastic
films of hard P V C, high pressure and low pressure polyethylene, polystyrene
and poly (methyl) methacrylate. Films of the polymer containing up to 0.5%
of u.v. absorbers were placed in contact for 10 days at $45^{\circ}C$ with water, 3%
acetic acid, 15%, 50% and 96% ethanol, heptane and sunflower seed oil, i.e. the
standard extractants of the Food and Drug Administration. Semi-quantitative
analyses for the extracted absorbers were carried out by thin-layer chromatography
on silica gel with cyclohexan e - acetic acid (4:1) or heptane - $CHCl_3$ (4:1)
as developing solvent. Hydroxybenzophenones were determined spectrophoto-
metrically at 290nm after evaporating the extract to dryness and dissolving
the residue in 96% ethanol. For hydroxyphenylbenzotriazoles, the dry residue
was dissolved in electrolyte (3ml of a solution containing 160ml of benzene
and 120ml of 5N-perchloric acid, 40ml of water and ethanol to 1 litre) and the
concentration was determined polarographically ($E_{\frac{1}{2}}$ = -1.45V).

Chapter 5

Determination of Specific Types of Additives in Aqueous and Alcoholic Extractants

5.1 PVC Plasticisers in Food

Wildbrett et al[11,12] have developed schemes for the measurement of the extractability of monomeric phthalate ester and C_{10}/C_{20} alkane phenyl sulphonates from PVC containers into milk. After leaving raw milk at 38° for 4 hours in contact with poly (vinyl chloride) tubing containing bis(2-ethylhexyl) phthalate or phenol or cresol alkanesulphonate, the respective plasticiser was determined. Schemes are described for separation and hydrolysis of the phthalic acid ester, with spectrophotometric determination at 284nm of the liberated phthalic acid, and for the separation and saponification of the alkanesulphonic acid ester and for spectrophotometric determination at 470nm of the liberated phenol or cresol after coupling with diazotised nitroaniline and addition of sodium carbonate solution.

These methods are applicable to the determination of dibutyl and di-isononyl phthalates, and of the C_{10} to C_{20} alkanesulphonates of phenol or cresol.

Wildbrett et al[12] also describe a scheme of analysis for the determination of milk fat in plastics, involving extraction with ethyl ether, saponification, isolation of glycerol, oxidation of the glycerol to formaldehyde and determination of formaldehyde with chromotropic acid.

For the determination of the extractability of phthalate esters from soft PVC Wildbrett et al[13] acidify the extract with hydrochloric acid, extract with light petroleum and dry the extract over anhydrous sodium sulphate, then evaporate in a rotary vacuum evaporator. The residue is dissolved in ethanol and the extinction measured at 274nm. A calibration graph is prepared with standard solution of bis-(2-ethylhexyl) phthalate. A scheme of analysis is also given for the isolation and determination of alkanesulphonate esters of phenol and cresols in the cleansing solution; it involves extraction and saponification of the esters and determination of phenol and cresols by reaction with diazotised 4-nitroaniline and measurement of the extinction at 470nm.

5.2 Organic Volatiles and Monomers in British Plastics Federation and Food and Drug Administration Extractants

Determination of acrylonitrile monomer. The procedures described below are based on cathode-ray polarography of a solution of the extractant in 0.02M

aqueous tetramethyl ammonium iodide. Polarographic cell solutions were
prepared by mixing 1ml of 0.2M aqueous base–distilled-water extractant.
The results obtained by polarography of 0.02M aqueous base–electolyte
solutions (start potential of –1.8 volts) showed that it is possible with
either the cathodic direct or the cathodic derivative circuits to determine
down to 1 ppm of acrylonitrile monomer in the distilled-water extractant.
Confirming the conclusions of Bird and Hale[14] and Daues and Hammer[15] it was
found that the presence in the cell solution of dissolved oxygen did not
interfere in the polarographic determination of acrylonitrile in the range
–1.8 to –2.3 volts.

Liquids obtained in extractability tests on styrene–acrylonitrile copolymers
also usually contain a small amount of styrene monomer besides acrylonitrile
monomer. It has been shown that the presence of up to 500ppm of styrene
monomer in the test solution does not interfere in the determination of
acrylonitrile in aqueous solutions.

Determination of acrylonitrile in aqueous-ethanol extractants. To 9ml of
each ethanol-water mixture containing 50ppm of added acrylonitrile was added
1ml of 0.2M tetramethylammonium iodide base-electrolyte solution. Reagent
blank solutions were also prepared by mixing 9ml of appropriate acrylonitrile
free ethanol-water mixture with 1ml of 0.2M base electrolyte. These samples
and blank solutions were examined polarographically at a start potential of
–1.8 volts and the peak currents occurring at the acrylonitrile maximum
were noted. The influence of the ethanol content of the extraction liquid
on the peak current obtained with 50ppm of acrylonitrile (corrected for the
peak current of the reagent blank solution) is shown in Fig.16. It is
seen that lower peak currents are obtained as the alcohol content of the test
solution increases from zero to 50%, i.e. the procedure for determining
acrylonitrile becomes rather less sensitive as the alcohol content of the
extraction liquid is increased. Acrylonitrile could be reproducibly determined,
however, in amounts down to 1ppm in all the alcohol solutions.

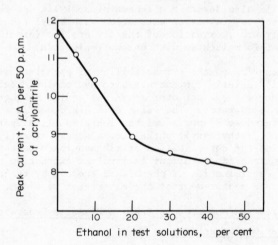

FIG.16 Graph of peak current versus ethanol concentration of test solution for
        50ppm of acrylonitrile in aqueous ethanol solutions containing 0.02M
        tetramethylammonium iodide base electrolyte.

Determination of acrylonitrile monomer in the 6% hydrochloric acid and the 5% sodium carbonate extractants. Direct polarography of synthetic solutions of acrylonitrile in the 6% hydrochloric acid and in the 5% sodium carbonate extractants is not possible as both extractants produced interfering waves in the acrylonitrile polarogram. Also, when tetramethylammonium iodide was added to the 6% hydrochloric acid extractant, the quaternary salt decomposed and free iodine was liberated.

The applicability of the azeotropic-distillation procedure described by Daues and Hamner[15] for separating acrylonitrile monomer from interfering impurities before polarography was examined. In this procedure the aqueous sample is distilled in the presence of a mixture of methanol and aqueous sulphuric acid. The methanol-acrylonitrile azeotrope, boiling at $61.4^{\circ}C$, distils first from this mixture and thus the acrylonitrile is recovered in the initial distillate.

The azeotropic-distillation procedure was tested by using a synthetic solution of acrylonitrile in water that had been shown by direct polarographic analysis to contain 0.75ppm of acrylonitrile. A measured volume (500ml) of this solution, ie.e 0.375mg of acrylonitrile, together with 5ml of concentrated sulphuric acid, 25ml of methanol and 0.1g of 2,4-dinitrophenyl-hydrazine (to destroy carbonyl compounds) was transferred to a round-bottomed flask fitted with a lagged glass column packed with $\frac{1}{8}$-inch helices and a reflux head. This mixture was distilled for 1 hour under total reflux and then three 4-ml portions of the methanol distillate were collected in separate 10-ml calibrated flasks. Then 1ml of 0.2M tetramethylammonium iodide and 5ml of distilled water were added to each flask. The weight of acrylonitrile recovered from the three fractions was determined polarographically by making "standard additions" of a synthetic solution of acrylonitrile in a methanol-water (40 + 60) mixture to the cell solution. It can be seen from Table 5 (sample A) that approximately 90% of the 0.375mg of acrylonitrile monomer present in the original 500ml of water was recovered in the first two 4-ml methanol distillates. The somewhat low recovery of acrylonitrile might be due to a slight hydrolysis of this substance to ammonium acrylate under the acidic conditions used during azeotropic distillation.

Determination of acrylonitrile in 6% hydrochloric acid extractant. The methanol azeotropic- distillation procedure was also applied to a synthetic solution of acrylonitrile in 6% hydrochloric acid extractant. Polarographic analysis of the methanol-acrylonitrile azeotrope was not possible, however, owing to the presence of an appreciable amount of free acidity originating from the hydrochloric acid extractant, in the distillates, which interfered in the polarography of acrylonitrile. In a further experiment, a 6% hydrochloric acid solution of 47.3ppm of acrylonitrile was neutralised by the addition of a small excess of solid calcium oxide. Methanol and sulphuric acid were added and the azeotropic distillation continued as before. In can be seen from Table 5 (sample B) that under these conditions more than 90% of the added amount of acrylonitrile was recovered in the first 8ml of methanol distillate. A preliminary neutralisation with lime was incorporated, therefore, into the procedure for determining acrylonitrile in 6% hydrochloric acid extraction liquids. This procedure should also be applicable to the determination of acrylonitrile in the 3% aqueous acetic acid extractant recommended by the Food and Drug Administration[2,3].

Determination of acrylonitrile monomer in 5% sodium carbonate extractant. The results in Table 5 (samples C and D) show that above 80% of the added amount of acrylonitrile was recovered in the methanol distillate when the azeotropic-distillation procedure was applied to 5% sodium carbonate extractants

containing up to 72.4ppm of acrylonitrile monomer. The recoveries of
acrylonitrile in these experiments are lower than those obtained for the
distilled-water and 6% hydrochloric acid extractants. This may be due to
an increased amount of hydrolysis of acrylonitrile to ammonium acrylate
occurring during reflux in the presence of sodium sulphate, as this salt
will elevate the temperature at which the mixture boils during the
preliminary 1 hour reflux period. The azeotropic-distillation procedure is
also applicable to the 3% sodium hydrogen carbonate extractant recommended
by the Food and Drug Administration (USA).[2],[3]

TABLE 5

DETERMINATION OF ACRYLONITRILE IN DISTILLED-WATER, 6 PER CENT HYDROCHLORIC ACID AND
5 PER CENT SODIUM CARBONATE EXTRACTANTS AFTER AZEOTROPIC DISTILLATION WITH METHANOL

Sample	Composition of synthetic test solution used for azeotropic distillation		Volume of test solution used for azeotropic distillation, ml	Acrylonitrile added, μg (X)	Weight, in μg, of acrylonitrile in test solution					Recovery of acrylonitrile in first two fractions obtained by azeotropic distillation ($\frac{Y \times 100}{X}$) per cent. w/w
	Acrylonitrile, p.p.m. w/v	Solvent			Found by direct polarography of sample, μg	Found in distillates obtained by azeotropic distillation with methanol				
						1 (1st 4ml)	2 (2nd 4ml)	3 (3rd 4ml)	Total (Y)	
A	0.75	Distilled water	500	376	376	315	21	Nil	336	90
B	47.3	6 per cent. HCl	50(+ 3.5 g of calcium oxide)	2370	–	2250	93	Nil	2343	99
C	14.4	5 per cent Na$_2$CO$_3$	25	360	–	248	54	Nil	302	84
D	72.4	5 per cent Na$_2$CO$_3$	25	1810	–	1390	83	Nil	1473	82

Determination of acrylonitrile in light-liquid-paraffin extractant. The
possibility of aqueous extraction of acrylonitrile from the liquid paraffin
was examined. Various synthetic solutions of acrylonitrile in liquid paraffin
were extracted with two 250-ml portions of distilled water. The distilled-
water extracts were filtered into a 1-litre flask and an azeotropic distillation
with methanol made as described previously. The recoveries of acrylonitrile
obtained by this procedure for liquid-paraffin extractants containing up to
538ppm of acrylonitrile are shown in Table 6. In all these mixtures, the
recovery of acrylonitrile in the first 8ml of the methanol azeotrope was
within 5% of the amount known to be prssent. Duplicate recoveries obtained
in the azeotropic-distillation procedure are reasonably reproducible.

Procedures, based on these principles, involving extraction with water and
azeotropic distillation with methanol before polarography should also be
applicable to the n-heptane extractant recommended by the Food and Drug
Administration[2],[3] and also might be useful for the determination of acrylonitrile
in the Food and Drug Administration vegetable-oil extractants, provided that
these can be successfully extracted with water. Trials have not been made on
these particular extractants.

TABLE 6

DETERMINATION OF ACRYLONITRILE IN LIGHT LIQUID-PARAFFIN EXTRACTANT

Acrylonitrile content of the synthetic light liquid-paraffin sample solution for extraction with water, p.p.m. w/w	Weight of light liquid-paraffin sample extracted with 2 X 250 ml of water, g	Weight of acrylonitrile present in light liquid-paraffin test solution, μg (X)	Weight, in μg, of acrylonitrile recovered in fractions of azeotropic distillation				Mean recovery of acrylonitrile in first two fractions obtained by azeotropic distillation ($\frac{Y \times 100}{X}$), per cent. w/w
			1 (1st 4 ml)	2 (2nd 4 ml)	3 (3rd 4 ml)	Total (Y)	
538	10	5380	(*i*) 4940	350	Nil	5290	99
			(*ii*) 4980	370	Nil	5350	
297	20	5940	5160	460	Nil	5620	95
34	200	6800	(*i*) 7220	Nil	Nil	7220	103
			(*ii*) 6840	Nil	Nil	6840	
11.1	9	100	(*i*) 96	2	Nil	98	98
			(*ii*) 96	2	Nil	98	

Detailed procedures for determining acrylonitrile monomer in the various extractants are described below:

Apparatus

Cathode-ray polarograph - K1000. Complete with stand for dropping mercury electrode, polarographic cells (10ml) and thermostatted (at 25°C) water-bath, supplied by Southern Analytical Ltd., Frimley Road, Camberley, Surrey, England.

Agla mictometer syringe - Capable of delivering 0.01ml with an accuracy of 0.0002ml, available from Burroughs Wellcome & Co., London.

Calibrated glassware - Pipettes, measuring cylinders and 10ml calibrated flasks.

Apparatus for azeotropic distillation with methanol - Connect a 1-litre round-bottomed flask (B24 neck) to a 60 x 1.8cm column packed with ¼-inch glass helices. Connect a reflux head, as described by Daues and Hammer[28] fitted with side-arm, condenser and stopcock, to the top of the column. Stand the round-bottomed flask, surrounded in aluminium foil, in an electric mantle. Wind an electric heating tape round the column and stand the whole apparatus in a draft-free area to prevent bumping during distillation.

Reagents

Methanol - Carbonyl-free. Heat 2 litres of methanol under reflux for 3 hours with 20g of aluminium powder and 50g of potassium hydroxide. Distil off the methanol into a clean bottle.

Calcium oxide.

2,4-Dinitrophenylhydrazine - Pure.

Tetramethylammonium iodide base electrolyte, 0.2M - 4.025g per 100ml water.

Acrylonitrile monomer.

Separation of Acrylonitrile from Light Liquid-Paraffin and n-Heptane Extractants

Weigh an amount of extractant containing between 0.001 and 0.01g of acrylonitrile into a clean 1-litre separating funnel. Into a further separating funnel, weigh the same amount of the blank extractant that has not been brought into contact with the plastic under test. Into each funnel pour 250ml of water. Stopper the funnels and shake the contents thoroughly. When the two phases have separated, filter the lower aqueous phase through two layers of Whatman No.40 filter-paper into a 1-litre round-bottomed flask. Extract the organic phase with a further 250ml of water and combine the aqueous extracts. As soon as possible after this extraction procedure, carry out an azeotropic distillation of the aqueous extracts with methanol as described below.

Determination of Acrylonitrile in Extractants.

Distilled water, 6% hydrochloric acid, 5% sodium carbonate, 3% sodium hydrogen carbonate and aqueous extract of light liquid-paraffin or n-heptane - Into a 1-litre round-bottomed flask transfer a volume of the plastic-extraction liquid containing between 0.001 and 0.01g of acrylonitrile. Into a further 1-litre flask transfer the same volume of the b lank extracti on liquid. Into each flask introduce distilled water to make the volume up to 500ml. To the 6% w/v hydrochloric acid extractant only, add a slight excess of calcium oxide (3.5g of calcium oxide per 50ml of 6% w/v hydrochloric acid is sufficient). To the 5% sodium carbonate and the 3% sodium hydrogen carbonate extractants only, add sufficient concentrated sulphuric a cid to neutralise the alkali present. To all extractants add 5ml of concentrated sulphuric acid, 25ml of redistilled carbonyl-free methanol, 0.1g of 2,4-dinitrophenylhydrazine and a few glass beads. Place the two flasks in 1-litre electric mantles and connect to each flask a 60mm column packed with ⅛-inch glass helices and a reflux head. Turn the stopcock on the reflux head to total reflux and turn on the water supply to the condenser on the reflux head. Set the voltage of the heating tape on the column to bring the column to about $10^{o}C$ above room temperature. Commence heating the flasks and leave them to equilibrate for 1 hour after methanol starts to condense at the reflux head.

After the 1 hour reflux period, transfer by pipette 2ml of 0.2M tetramethyl-ammonium iodide base electrolyte and 10ml of water into each of two dry 25ml stoppered graduated cylinders. Place one of these cylinders at the outlet of the reflux head and open the stopcock to provide a reflux ratio of approximately 1 to 1. Allow methanol to distil into the cylinder at a rate of approximately 1ml per minute, until the volume of solution reaches the 20ml mark. Immediately examine the distillates polarographically as described below. It has been shown that up to 0.02g of acrylonitrile in the distillation-flask charge is recovered in the first 8ml of methanol-acrylonitrile azeotrope. Completeness of recovery of acrylonitrile in this distillate can be checked by collecting a further 4ml of distillate in a 10ml graduated cylinder (containing 1ml of 0.2M tetramethylammonium iodide and 5ml of distilled water). Polarography of the solution shows whether any acrylonitrile is present in the second distillate. If acrylonitrile is found in this distillate then it should be included in the reported analytical result.

When the K1000 polarograph is used for the analysis, use a dropping mercury electrode and a mercury-pool reference electrode on the cathodic direct circuit. Transfer by pipette 5ml of sample solution from the 25ml cylinder

into a polarograph cell and immerse the cell in the constant-temperature tank
of the cathode-ray polarograph. Lower the dropping mercury electrode system
over this cell and insert the anode connection into the side-arm of the
polarographic cell. If the approximate concentration of monomer in the
polarographic cell solution is known, set the instrument to the appropriate
sensitivity setting at a start potential of -1.8volts. If the composition
of the solution is unknown, then adjust the polarograph to its maximum
sensitivity setting and move the "X-shift" control and the "Y-shift" control
until the light spot on the graticule of the cathode-ray tube commences its
horizontal sweep at the origin of axes at the left of the graticule. Repeat
this operation at different sensitivity settings until the polarographic wave
is visible on the graticule.

Read off from the graticule the maximum height of the peak, and note the
voltage, V, at which this maximum polarographic reading occurs. Transfer
by pipette a further 5ml of solution from the 25ml graduated cylinder into
a dry 25ml beaker and into this solution deliver a suitable "standard
addition" of a solution of acrylonitrile in a methanol-water (40+60,v/v)
mixture (by using a horizontally held Agla micrometer syringe for delivery).
To avoid dilution errors, limit the volume of the "standard addition" added
to less than 0.05ml. Mix the contents of the beaker and pour them into a
dry polarographic cell. Note the height of the acrylonitrile wave at V volts.
Adjust the instrument to obtain the azeotropic-distillation blank wave on
the graticule. Measure the blank peak height corresponding to V volts.

Aqueous ethanol – The azeotropic-distillation procedure cannot be applied to
this alcoholic extraction liquid. Transfer 16ml of the aqueous alcohol
plastic-extraction liquid and 16ml of the blank alcoholic extraction liquid
into two 25ml stoppered graduated cylinders. To each cylinder add 2ml of
0.2M tetramethylammonium iodide and 2ml of distilled water and mix. Examine
these solutions polarographically as described above.

Calculation of the acrylonitrile contents of the extractants. The amount of
acrylonitrile in the plastic-extraction liquid, ppm w/v, is given by:

$$\frac{20 \times A \times 10^6}{5 \times S} \left[\frac{h_1 S_1 - h_3 S_3}{h_2 S_2 - h_1 S_1} \right]$$

(assuming that the methanolic azeotropic distillate is made up to 20ml and
that 5ml of this solution is used for polarography), where:

S	= volume, in ml, of plastic-extraction liquid used in azeotropic distillation,
h_1	= peak height, in cm, of sample solution before the "standard addition",
h_2	= peak height, in cm, of sample solution after the "standard addition",
h_3	= peak height, in cm, obtained in the azeotropic-distillation blank determination,
S_1, S_2, S_3	are the corresponding instrument sensitivity settings (the products of h and S are known as peak currents, in μA) and
A	= weight, in g, of acrylonitrile present in volume of "standard addition", solution added to the cell solution.

Provided that a suitable sample size is taken for analysis, the azeotropic
distillation-polarographic procedure can be used for determining
acrylonitrile in extractants in concentrations down to 1ppm or a little
lower. Thus it is seen in Table 5 that approximately 90% of the added
amounts of acrylonitrile is recovered when the procedure is applied to
500ml of a 0.75ppm solution of acrylonitrile in the distilled-water extractant.
The method can be used for achieving a similar level of sensitivity in the
determination of acrylonitrile in the other aqueous alcoholic or oily
extractants for plastics recommended by the British Plastics Federation[1]
and the Food and Drug Administration[2,3]. This level of sensitivity is quite
adequate for the examination of extractants that have been brought into
contact with styrene-acrylonitrile copolymers under the British Plastics
Federation and Food and Drug Administration extractability-test conditions.

Actual extraction liquids obtained in extractability tests made on various
styrene-acrylonitrile copolymers have been found by the described procedures
to contain from less than 10ppm up to 200ppm of acrylonitrile. The amount
of acrylonitrile monomer found in the extraction liquids depends, of course,
on the extent to which this monomer is removed from the plastic during the
manufacturing process.

It is advisable to analyse an extraction liquid for acrylonitrile as soon
as possible after the completion of the extractability tests. This is because
a slow hydrolysis of acrylonitrile to acrylamide or ammonium acrylate occurs
on standing, especially in acidic or alkaline extractants. Consequently,
low acrylonitrile contents are obtained by the polarographic method. Thus,
on analysis immediately after the extraction test, a 6% hyrochloric acid
extractant was found to contain 110ppm of acrylonitrile. Analysis of the
same sample two months later showed that the acrylonitrile content had
decreased to 75ppm owing to the hydrolysis.

Determination of styrene monomer and other volatiles in polystyrene. Conventional
and modified grades of polystyrene contain low concentrations of residual
styrene monomer left in from the manufacturing process. In addition to
monomer, the polymer might contain other aromatic volatiles such as ethyl
benzene , cumene etc., which originate as impurities in the styrene charge-
stock. In the case of grades of polystyrene used for foodstuff or beverage
packaging applications, some transfer will occur of these volatiles from the
container to its contents with consequent risk of contamination and tainting
of the packaged commodity.

In order to measure the extent to which the aromatic polystyrene volatiles
migrate from a polymer, gas chromatography can be used to determine low
concentrations of these substances in the aqueous and alcoholic British
Plastics Federation extractants. The gas chromatographic separation column
comprised polyethylene glycol 20,000 (Carbowax 15-20M) supported on Celite
(60-72mesh), and detection was achieved using a flame ionisation detector
which has the advantage of high sensitivity and freedom from interference by
water in the sample. The instrumental conditions are those of Shapras and
Claver[16] in which a 5µl sample is injected into a separation system comprising
two columns in series consisting of a 10ft × ½inOD column of Tween 81 (20%)
an Chromosorb W (30-60mesh) and Resoflex 446 (10%) on Chromosorb W (30-60mesh)
using a hydrogen flame detector to achieve the desired sensitivity and
nitrogen (25ml/mm) as carrier gas. Figure 17 shows the chromatogram obtained
with synthetic solutions in the aqueous and an alcoholic British Plastics
Federation extractant of various aromatic volatiles likely to occur in the
polystyrene. The extractants are injected directly into the gas
chromatograph (the olive oil or liquid paraffin extractants cannot be
injected directly into the gas chromatographic column). Mixtures of benzene,

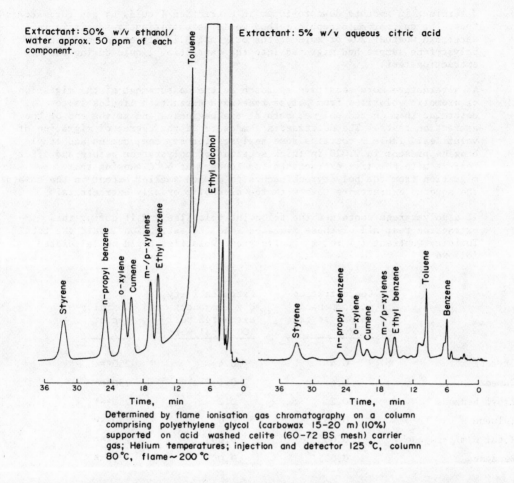

Extractant: 50% w/v ethanol/ water approx. 50 ppm of each component.

Extractant: 5% w/v aqueous citric acid

Determined by flame ionisation gas chromatography on a column comprising polyethylene glycol (carbowax 15-20 m) (10%) supported on acid washed celite (60-72 BS mesh) carrier gas; Helium temperatures; injection and detector 125 °C, column 80 °C, flame ~ 200 °C

FIG.17   Gas chromatographic determination of aromatic volatiles in polystyrene extraction liquids.

toluene, ethyl benzene, n-propyl benzene, o-xylene, cumene, m/p-xylene and styrene monomer were resolved from each other and could each be detected in amounts down to approximately 10ppm.

To obtain quantitative determinations of aromatic volatiles in the extraction liquids it is necessary to adopt the standard gas chromatographic technique of incorporating into the extractant a known concentration of a miscible internal standard substance which has a different retention time to any of the sample components.

Under the extractability test conditions prescribed by the British Plastics Federation for plastic test pieces of less than 0.020 in thickness, the plastic and the extractant are contacted under standard test conditions at a ratio of 1cm³ plastic volume to 20ml extractant[1].   Thus if a polystyrene test piece contained 0.1% styrene monomer and this completely migrated into the extractant during the test, then at the end of the extraction test the extractant would contain approximately 5 0ppm monomer.   Styrene monomer can be determined in amounts down to 10ppm in extraction liquids by gas chromatography. Thus, the gas chromatographic method would be sufficiently sensitive to ascertain whether 20% or more of the original 0.1% styrene monomer in the polystyrene sample had migrated into the extraction liquid during the extraction test.

An alternative more sensitive approach to the measurement of the migration of aromatic volatiles from polystyrene into extraction liquids is to determine them in the polymer both at the beginning and at the end of the extraction tests. The decrease is a measure of the degree of migration of volatiles. Table 7 contains some analyses for styrene, cumene and ethyl benzene present in 0.020 in thick sections of polystyrene before and after contact with the five extractants for 10 days at $60^{\circ}C$ showing that migration from the polystyrene occurs to a much smaller extent in the case of the aqueous extractants than with the alcoholic or oily extractants.

If a polystyrene contained the following volatiles and if during the extraction test all of these migrated into the extraction liquid the total Toxicity Quotient (Q) for the polystyrene volatiles could be calculated as follows:

	Concentration of component in polystyrene % w/w	Extractability, E g component extracted per 100ml polymer*	Toxicity factor (T)
Styrene	0.4	0.4	250**
Cumene	0.4	0.4	250***
Ethyl benzene	0.2	0.2	250***
Toluene	0.05	0.05	250***
Total o/m/p-xylene	0.005	0.005	250***
Benzene	0.005	0.005	1***

* Assuming that polymer has a density of unity and that the additives completely migrate from the polymer during the extraction test.

** Taken from British Plastics Federation Second Toxicity Report[1]

*** Assumed values if $Q = \Sigma \frac{E \times 1000}{T}$

Then Q (for the polystyrene components excluding benzene) = 4.2

Q (for the 0.005% (50ppm) benzene)   = 5.0

Q (for total migrated polymer components)   = 9.2

These data show that, based on the above assumption regarding toxicity factors, 50 to 100ppm extractable benzene in the polymer would render the polymer unacceptable for food packaging applications (i.e. Q>10). Small concentrations of benzene have been detected occasionally in polystyrene. Considerably higher concentrations of extractable aromatics other than benzene can be tolerated in the polymer. Usually, however, in the case of food or beverage packaging grades of polystyrene, it is necessary to reduce the level of all aromatics to a very low level as, in addition to

toxicity considerations, food tainting by migrated polymer volatiles is an
additional factor governing the acceptability of a polymer in this field.

TABLE 7

Migration of aromatic volatiles from 0.020 in thick

polystyrene sections in the British Plastics

Federation extractants

Aromatics determined in polystyrene[a], % w/w

Extraction Liquid	Styrene		Cumene		Ethyl benzene	
	Before extraction	After extraction	Before extraction	After extraction	Before extraction	After extraction
Distilled water	0.14	0.13	0.012	0.012	0.016	0.015
5% sodium carbonate	0.13	0.12	0.012	0.013	0.014	0.015
5% citric acid	0.13	0.12	0.012	0.011	0.013	0.015
50% ethyl alcohol: water	0.12	0.09	0.012	0.011	0.015	0.013
Liquid paraffin	0.10	0.02	0.011	0.004	0.014	0.003

(a) 2g polystyrene contacted with 100ml extraction liquid

5.3 Determination of Organotin Stabilizers in Non-fatty Simulents and Foods, and in Sunflower Seed Cooking Oil

A good example of the application of elemental analysis to the analysis of
extractants and foods after contact with plastics is the determination of
organotin compounds in these materials via their catechol-violet complex.

Adcock and Hope[17] have developed the method, described below, for the
determination of dioctyltin S,S' bis-(iso-octylmercaptoacetate) as tin in the range
0.2-1.6μg in vinegar and orange drink. The American Food and Drugs
Administration Regulations permit the presence in certain foodstuffs, as a
result of migration, of two organotin compounds, namely, di-octyltin SS'-
bis-(iso-octylmercaptoacetate) and di-octyltin maleate polymer. The concentration
of either, or any combination of both, may not exceed 1ppm which represents
0.158 or 0.259ppm of tin (as organotin), respectively, in the foodstuff.
Convenience and necessity may limit the amount of foodstuffs available for
analysis to, say, 5g. In such a situation a procedure for the determination
of about 0.75μg of tin is essential.

Method
Preparation of tin calibration curve
Reagents and Materials
All reagents should be of analytical-reagent grade.

Water, de-ionised
Sulphuric acid, sp.gr. 1.84
Sulphuric acid, N
Hydrochloric acid, sp.gr. 1.18
Dilute hydrochloric acid (1+2.2) - Dilute hydrochloric acid (sp.gr. 1.18)
   appropriately with water
Catechol violet, 0.05% w/v, aqueous - Prepare fresh weekly
Sodium acetate trihydrate - sodium hydroxide solution - Prepare a solution
   containing 40g of sodium acetate trihydrate and 8.3g of sodium hydroxide in
   250ml. Check this solution by adding 1ml to a mixture of 0.3ml of N
   sulphuric acid, 0.9ml of water, 0.4ml of dilute hydrochloric acid and 0.4ml
   of catechol violet solution. If the resultant solution does not have a pH
   of 3.8, adjust the sodium acetate-sodium hydroxide solution by adding a
   solution of sodium acetate of equal concentration but with higher or lower
   sodium hydroxide concentration as necessary. (The difference in pH between
   two mixed solutions, one prepared with a sodium acetate-sodium hydroxide
   solution containing 3g of sodium hydroxide per 250ml of solution and the
   other with an acetate-hydroxide solution containing 9g of sodium hydroxide
   per 250ml, is about 0.2pH unit).
Sodium acetate trihydrate-hydrochloric acid solution - Prepare a 20% w/v
   aqueous solution of sodium acetate trihydrate and add sufficient hydrochloric
   acid to produce a pH of 3.8.
Asbestos fibres - Treat Gooch asbestos as follows. Slurry the asbestos with a
   dilute aqueous solution of the selected surface-active agent, by using a
   high speed mixer. Add distilled water to produce a dilute suspension of
   fibres, and allow all but the "fines" to settle. Decant. Repeat the
   diluting and decanting steps twice. Collect the asbestos on a Buchner
   funnel and wash it with distilled water until it is free from surface-active
   agent. Dry the asbestos at 105°C.
Fibrous cellulose powder - A suitable column-chromatographic grade, i.e.
   powder that disperses readily in aqueous solutions, settles freely and
   gives columns with high flow-rates, besides possessing adequate adsorptive
   capacity for the tin-catechol violet complex.
Surface-active agent, non-ionic or anionic, 0.5% v/v aqueous solution -
   Tergitol NPX (from B.D.H. Chemicals Ltd.) has been found satisfactory.
Tin(IV) stock solution - Dissolve 0.1000g of pure tin in 20ml of sulphuric
   acid, sp.gr. 1.84, by heating until fumes appear. Cool cautiously dilute
   with 150ml of water and cool again. Ad 65ml of sulphuric acid, sp.gr. 1.84
   cool and transfer to a 500ml calibrated flask. Dilute to the mark with
   water (1ml of solution ≡ 200µg of tin).
Tin(IV) dilute standard solution - Dilute 1.0ml of tin (IV) stock solution
   with 30ml of N sulphuric acid to 100ml. Prepare just before use (1ml of
   solution ≡ 2µg of tin).

Transfer to a series of 10ml beakers by pipette (or small-capacity burette),
volumes of dilute standard tin solution to cover the whole or a suitable
part of the range 0 to 1.6µg of tin. Evaporate the solutions to dryness, first
by heating on a steam bath and finally by heating in a muffle furnace at
300°C until no sulphuric acid remains. Cool the beakers. Treat each as
follows: add 0.3ml of N sulphuric acid and warm on a steam bath. With the aid
of a glass rod and by rotation of the beaker, ensure that the whole of the
inside of the beaker is wetted with warm acid. Allow the solution to evaporate
to the fullest extent that steam bath heating conditions permit. Cool. Add
in order, without delay between each addition but with adequate mixing after
each addition, 0.9ml of water, 0.4ml of dilute hydrochloric acid, 0.4ml of
catechol violet solution and 1.0 ml of sodium acetate-sodium hydroxide
solution.   Set aside for 3 hours.

Prepare asbestos or cellulose powder columns, one for use with each beaker, as
follows: lightly plug with cottonwool, to a distance of about 5mm, the end of
a piece of glass tubing of about 4mm i.d. and not less than 150mm long.
Trim the plug so that no cottonwool fibres protrude. Slurry 0.10g of
asbestos or 0.15g of cellulose powder with a few millilitres of sodium
acetate-hydrochloric acid solution and transfer all of the slurry to the
plugged tube, by using additional solution as required. Allow the powder
to settle and pack as freely as possible, disturbing it only if it becomes
necessary to release any trapped air bubbles. When the excess of solution
has drained through, the column is ready for use. The internal volume of the
tubing above the column should be not less than 1.5ml.

With a Pasteur pipette, transfer to the top of the column the whole of the
solution that has been allowed to stand for 3 hours. Wash the 10ml beaker
with about 1.5ml of sodium acetate-hydrochloric acid solution and transfer
the whole on to the column as soon as there is no more coloured solution above
it. Allow the column to drain and remove, by touching any hanging drop.
Reject all column effluents. Without further delay add 1.5ml of surface-active
agent solution to the column to elute the tin-catechol violet complex and
collect all of the 1.5ml of eluate. With surface-active agent solution in a
reference cell measure the optical density of the eluate in a 20mm path
micro cell, at the wavelength appropriate for the complex in the surface-
active agent chosen (with Tergitol, NPX, about 570nm). Construct a graph for
amount of tin versus optical density.

Determination of dioctyltin S,S' bis-(iso-octylmercaptoacetate) in vinegar and
orange drink. The tin stabiliser can be extracted from these foodstuffs by
various chlorinated solvents and hydrocarbons, but well defined separation of
solvent and foodstuff, after shaking them together to effect extraction, is
not readily achieved even by centrifuging the mixture. Continuous extraction
in an extractor of the type shown in Fig. 18a avoids this difficulty.
Extraction with petroleum spirit is slower, but gives a cleaner extract than
extraction with chlorinated solvents (for which a differently designed
extractor was used).

Dilute solutions of stabiliser readily deposit organotin compounds on the
surfaces of their containers. Consequently, when for the purpose of
checking the recovery obtainable by a proposed analytical procedure a small
amount of a dilute solution of stabiliser is added to a foodstuff, the weight
of stabiliser then present in that solution must be determined. It cannot
be calculated from the weight of stabiliser used for making the solution.

Organotin compounds deposited on the surface of the extraction flask during
continuous extraction cannot readily be removed with simple common solvents,
but their removal can be effected with a dilute solution of formic acid in,
say, diethylether. A 2% formic acid (100%) solution in ether does not rapidly
decompose the stabiliser. With higher concentrations the decomposition risk
is increased.

Newman and Jones[18], Suk and Malat[19] and Ross and White[20] list aluminium,
gallium, indium, titanium, zirconium, thorium, antimony, bismuth, molybdenum,
tungsten and iron as interfering species at the pH used for determining tin.
Of these species, only aluminium and iron are likely to be present in foodstuffs, and these are separated from the mercaptoacetate organotin stabiliser
by paper chromatography, with chloroform as developing solvent. Inorganic
tin compounds are also separated from the stabiliser under the same conditions
The stabiliser travels in or just behind the solvent front. By double

chromatographic development and the use of chromatographic paper cut to a special shape (Fig.18b) the stabiliser present in a few millilitres of petroleum spirit extract can be isolated within a paper area of 1 to 2cm .

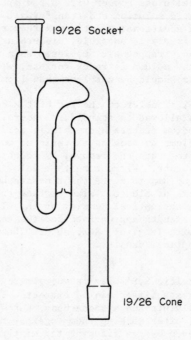

FIG.18a Apparatus for continuous extraction (approx 1/4 actual size).

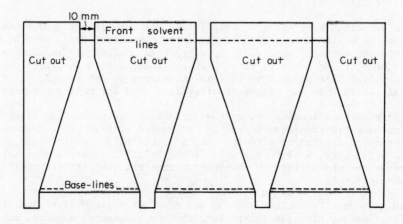

FIG.18b Chromatographic paper cut to shape (approx 1/3 actual size)

The area occupied by stabiliser can be established by spraying with
4-(2-pyridylazo)-resorcinol disodium salt (PAR), which produces a pink area
on a yellow background.

The paper plus stabiliser can be oxidised with sulphuric acid-hydrogen peroxide
mixture and the resulting solution evaporated to dryness at 300°C, to give a
tin sulphate residue for which the previously described method for tin
determination is appropriate.

Reagents and Apparatus

Petroleum spirit, boiling range 60° to 80°C - Glass-distilled to minimise
   metallic contamination.
Formic adid, 98 to 100% - For preparation of a 2% v/v solution in ether.
Diethyl ether
Chloroform
4-(2-Pryidylazo) resorcinol, disodium salt (PAR), 0.5% v/v solution in ethanol
Sulphuric acid, approximately 72% w/v - Dilute 64ml of concentrated acid,
   sp.gr. 1.98 to 100ml.
Micro Kjeldahl flasks - Working capacity 0.5 to 0.7ml. See procedure for
   orange drink extracts.
Continuous extractor - For extracting solvents lighter than the sample to be
   extracted. Sample capacity 5ml.
Chromatographic paper - Whatman No.1 or equivalent.
Pasteur pipette - The body consists of normal diameter glass tubing, joined
   to capillary tubing drawn out to produce the top of the pipette.
Hair dryer or equivalent - This is used as a source of clean cold air.

Procedure

Extract 5ml of vinegar (or orange drink) continuously with petroleum spirit
for 2 hours, maintaining as fast a rate of extraction as possible.
Concentrate the extract to about 1ml, preferably at about 30°C, but do not
allow it to evaporate to dryness.

Cut chromatographic paper to the shape shown in Fig.18b. With a capillary-
ended Pasteur pipette, apply the concentrated extract to the base-line.
Simultaneously, blow clean cold air on to the base-line area (preferably
on to the underside of the paper) to minimise spread of the extract and to
speed its evaporation. Continue blowing air until the paper is dry. Wash
the extraction flask with two 0.2ml portions of formic acid-ether solution and
transfer the washings in a similar way to the base-line. Air dry the paper
until it is substantially free from the smell of formic acid.

Develop the chromatogram with chloroform to the pre-drawn solvent front line.
Dry the chromatogram in air and carry out a second development. After again
removing the chloroform by exposure to air, spray the chromatogram with
4-(2-pyridylazo)resorcinol solution.The pink area at the solvent front contains
the stabiliser. Cut out this area.

Vinegar extracts. For these extracts place the cut-out paper in a 10ml
beaker. Add 0.5ml of 75% w/w sulphuric acid and warm on a steam-bath to
disperse, and lightly char the paper. Add two drops of Aristar hydrogen
peroxide and allow them to react. Add further peroxide, a few drops at a
time as necessary, to produce a colourless solution. Evaporate the solution
first to as small a volume as possible at 105°C, then to dryness at 300°C.

(If the solution becomes coloured during evaporation, cool the beaker
slightly, add 1 drop of peroxide and after a few minutes continue the
evaporation). For the determination of the tin in the residue in the beaker,
proceed as given under Preparation of calibration graph from "Cool the
beakers. Treat each as follows ... "

Orange drink extracts. In these extracts orange oil will be present in the
cut-out paper. This reacts too vigorously with sulphuric acid-hydrogen
peroxide for this treatment to be conducted in an open beaker without risk
of loss by splashing. Hence, carry out the oxidation in a micro Kjeldahl
flask (made by blowing a bulb at the end of a 12×100mm Pyrex test-tube).
Continue treatment until a colourless solution is maintained while sulphuric
acid fumes are being driven off. Transfer the cooled solution to a 10ml
beaker with a Pasteur pipette. Wash the flask and pipette with two 0.2ml
portions of N sulphuric acid and add the washings to the 10ml beaker.
Evaporate the solution at 105°C, then heat to dryness at 300°C, and proceed
to the determination of tin as given under Preparation of calibration graph
from "Cool the beakers. Treat each as follows ... "

Koch and Figge[21] studied the migration of organotin stabilisers such as
bis (2-ethylhexyloxycarbonyl)methylthio dioctyltin from PVC bottles into beer.
After storage of beer for 8 weeks at 20° in bottles stabilised with 1.13% of
bis- (2-ethylhexyloxycarbonyl)methylthio dioctyltin, it was treated with
sulphuric acid - nitric acid and tin was determined with catechol violet by
the method of Newman and Jones[18].

The tin was also determined by measurement of radioactivity after storage
of beer in bottles stabilised with (C-labelled bis [(2-ethylhexyloxycarbonyl)
methylthio]dioctyltin. Only 1.7µg of Sn per litre was found; the F.D.A.
limit being 1mg per litre.

The isolation and determination of organotin compounds in vinegar and salad
oil after contact with stabilised hard PVC foil has also been studied by
Wiecorek[22]. Some foil samples were extracted under reflux, with pentane or
ethyl ether; other samples were left in contact with oil or vinegar for
periods up to 11 months. The organotin compounds in the solvent extracts
or in the oil (diluted with pentane) or a chloroform extract of the vinegar
were then adsorbed on to a column of Florisil (which was then washed with
hexane and ether, if necessary, to remove oil), eluted with chloroform-
acetic acid-ether (5:4:3) and separated by thin-layer chromatography[23].
In comparison with the amount of organotin compounds that migrates from the
foil into salad oil during storage for 11 months at room temperature, ether
extraction for 5 hours removes ≈830 times as much, but pentane extraction for
1 hour removes only about 20% of the amount. From 11.5 to 27µg of organically
bound tin per sq dm of foil was found to migrate into the oil during
11 months.

5.4 Determination of additives in extraction liquids via elemental analysis

Determination of additives via the determination of elements such as sulphur,
halogens, phosphorus and nitrogen, offers a further method of extractant
analysis, provided that the additives can first be quantitatively extracted
from a large volume of the liquid with a low-boiling organic solvent.
Conventional microchemical methods are available for determining these
elements with adequate sensitivity such that they are amenable to many
extractant analysis problems (Table 8).

Besides occurring in polymers in the form of additives, elements such as
chlorine, sulphur, nitrogen and phosporus can also occur in virgin polymers
in the form of impurities. Thus, virgin polystyrene might contain residual
concentrations of chlorine and phosphorus originating as potassium chloride
and inorganic phosphates added during polymerisation. High-density
polyolefins contain chlorine up to 600ppm (originating from catalysts) and
sulphur (up to 200ppm). During an extraction test these elements might
migrate to a small extent from the polymer and consequently interfere in
methods for determining polymer additives based on the determination of the
same element. Nevertheless, methods based on the determination of
elements can be useful, is being shown in the case of dilaurylthiodipropionate
(Chapter 7).

Metal-containing compounds are sometimes used in the formulation of plastics.
The British Plastics Federation in their Second Toxicity Report[1] has described
sensitive procedures for determining barium, cadmium, copper and lead in their
five representative extractants.

Sluzewska[24] has discussed the detection of organometallic stabilisers and the
migration thereof from PVC food containers. He uses thin-layer chromatography
for the detection of compounds of barium, cadmium, lead and zinc. The PVC
sample (10g) is cut into 1cm squares and soaked in saturated sodium nitrite
solution for 24 hours the squares are then extracted with 3% acetic acid
by boiling under reflux for 5 hours. The resulting extracts are boiled to
dryness and the residue dissolved in 5ml of concentrated hydrochloric acid,
which is again evaporated then dissolved in 5 ml 1 molar hydrochloric acid
and filtered. An aliquot of the filtrate is then applied to a 0.25mm thick
cellulose layer and the chromatogram developed with ethanol-propanol-acetic
acid-water (15:15:2:8) and the spots located with 1% aqueous sodium rhodizoate.
From 5 to 10µg of each metal can be detected in this way.

5.5   Use of labelled additives in extractability tests

The use of radioactive labelled additives has obvious attractions in studies
connected with the extractability of additives from plastics. In theory,
all that is necessary is to prepare the additive in a suitably labelled
form, determine its specific activity, incorporate a known amount of it in
the polymer and carry out the extraction test. Suitable counting carried
out on the extraction liquid and/or on the polymer enables the degree of
ad d itive migration into the extraction liquid to be determined. In
practice however the problem is not always as simple as this.

Some additives used in polymer, formulations are pure compounds whilst others
are complex mistures. If a realistic assessment is to be obtained of the
extractability of an additive from a plastic, then preparations of labelled
additives. must have an identical chemical composition to the commercial
products. Usually it is simpler to synthesise a chemically pure compound
with particular atoms labelled than it is to synthesise a specifically labelled
product which has exactly the same chemical composition as an impure commercial
material. For this reason the radiochemical approach is more attractive
in those cases involving a fairly pure additive than when the additive is
impure.

Obviously, the development of methods for determining additives is easier
in cases where no breakdown has occurred of the additive either during
polymer processing or during the polymer extraction test. Analysis for the
undegraded additive in the presence of its breakdown products is inevitably

TABLE 8

Methods of determination of traces of various elements in extraction liquids

Element	Procedure	Reference	Interferences
Sulphur	Low-boiling solvent extract (max. 30mg) evaporated onto a piece of filter paper and combusted in oxygen-filled flask over dilute hydrogen peroxide solution.	25,26	Chloride, fluoride phosphate, nitrogen, boron, and metals, all interfere
	Potentiometric titration of sulphuric acid with N/100 sodium hydroxide or photometric titration of sulphate with N/100 barium perchlorate.		Up to 2mg chlorine fluorine, nitrogen, boron and metals do not interfere in the determination of 1mg sulphur. Phosphorus (up to 2mg) interferes in the determination of sulphur (1mg), but this interference can be overcome using the procedure of Colson[25-27]
Chlorine (or bromine	Combustion as above.		
	Chloride titrated potentiometrically with N/100 silver nitrate in presence of nitric in presence of nitric acid and acetone		
Chlorine or bromine or iodine	Combustion as above.	27	Up to 8mg phosphorus, fluorine, sulphur, do not interfere in determination of 2mg chlorine.
	Halide titrated with mercuric nitrate		
Phosphorus	Low-boiling solvent extract evaporated on to a piece of filter paper and digested with sulphuric acid/perchloric acid	28	No interference by sulphur, ch orine, fluorine, nitrogen
	Digested diluted and ammonium vandate/ ammonium molybdate added. Yellow phosphovand-molybdate complex evaluated at 430nm.		

TABLE 8 continued

Element	Procedure	Reference	Interferences
Nitrogen	Low-boiling solvent extract evaporated on to a piece of filter paper and a Kjeldahl digestion carried out.	29	No interference by sulphur, halogens and phosphorus
	(a) Kjeldahl digest made alkaline and distilled into 4% boric acid. Ammonia estimated by acid titration.		
	(b) Spectrophotometric estimation at 630mμ of phenol-indophenol derivative.		
Fluorine	Low-boiling solvent extract evaporated onto a piece of filter paper and combusted in an oxygen filled flask over distilled water.	30	No interference by large excesses of sulphur chlorine, phosphorus and nitrogen
	Reacted with buffered alizarin complex/cerous nitrate, blue colour produced evaluated at 610nm.		
Silicon	Low-boiling solvent extract evaporated into gelatine capsule and combusted with sodium peroxide, sucrose and benzoic acid in 22ml capacity Parr Bomb.	31	No inteference by sulphur, halogens, phosphorus, nitrogen and boron.
	Solution adjusted to pH1.0 to 1.5 in presence of ammonium molybdate and the yellow silico-molybdic acid complex evaluated at 390nm.		
Boron	Low-boiling solvent extract evaporated into small ampoule and dissolved in acetone. Sample is digested with concentrated nitric acid in a sealed ampoule to convert organo boron compounds to boric acid.		No interference by chlorine and nitrogen.
	Digest dissolved in methyl alcohol and boron estimated flame-photometrically at 519.5nm.		

more complicated than is the case when degradation has not occurred. Before
adopting a radiochemical method for the estimation of additives in extractants
it is necessary to ascertain the degree of degradation of the additive. If
degradation has not occurred, simple counting of the extraction liquid and the
extracted polymer at the end of the extraction test will give reliable informati
on the degree of additive migration that has occurred. If, however, it can be
shown that the additive has appreciably degraded during processing and/or
the extraction test, then simple counting to total radioactivity in the
extractant and the polymer at the end of the extraction test is insufficient
and the radiochemical procedure must be suitably elaborated to distinguish
between the radioactive degraded and undegraded forms of the additive.
Unpublished work on the measurement of the extractability of Alromine RU 100
(a fatty acid-diethanolamine condensate) from polypropylene film, has
illustrated the types of difficulty encountered in applying radiochemical
methods to extractant analysis. Alromine RU 100 is an impure condensation
product of diethanolamine and a fatty acid. It degrades, partially, during
polymer processing and also hydrolyses extensively during extraction tests
with aqueous extractants. Thus, all the difficulties discussed above,
concerning application of the radiochemical procedure to extractability testing,
were encountered in the development of a method for determining this additive in
extractants.

Little work has been published of the use of labelled additives in the
measurement of migration into aqueous extraction liquids. A notable
exception is the work carried out by Koch and Figge[21] the measurement of
the migration of labelled di-n-octyltin-bis-(2-ethylhexylthioglycolate) from
PVC bottles into beer   (see Chapter 5.3). Labelled additives have, on the
other hand, been used extensively with studies of migration into fatty
extractants and foods and this is discussed further in Chapter 6.

Chapter 6

Determination of Additives in Edible Oils and Fatty Foodstuffs Extractants

6.1. Introductory discussion of extraction test

Whilst in most of the official regulations the simulents and extraction test conditions to be applied are practically the same in the case of aqueous, low-fat or fat-free foodstuffs, this is not so in the case of additive migration from plastics into fatty foodstuffs.

The direct quantitative determination of additives migrating from plastics into edible oils or fatty foodstuffs (Woggon and Uhde[32]) is extremely difficult even with the most sophisticated analytical techniques, and in some cases it may be impossible. Analytical procedures in which the migrated additives are concentrated or isolated from the fatty foodstuffs before their determination are tedious. Moreover they are inaccurate because of losses of material and they may even fail completely. Therefore, in order to determine the migrated additives quantitatively in an analytically suitable simulant, it is essential to simulate the natural migration into foodstuffs in appropriate model tests.

The fat simulants used in many countries are mainly simple organic solvents such as n-heptane (Food and Drug Administration, 1967 [3], Italian Ministry of Health, 1963[33], diethyl ether (Franck[34]) and paraffin oil (British Plastics Federation[1]), substances completely different in chemical structure from the triglycerides of edible oils Alternatively, edible oils, such as olive oil (British Plastics Federation[1]), coconut oil (Franck[34]) and others have been proposed as test fats without any allowance being made for the analytical difficulties. However, as Figge[31] has pointed out, since edible oils and fats, as well as other fatty foodstuffs, are increasingly marketed in plastics packages, there is a growing demand for a standard method for the simulation of natural migration phenomena.

Detailed data on the extraction capacities of these fat simulants in comparison with the actual migration of additives from plastics into fatty food have been elaborated by Figge[36 37 38 39], Eder and Piater,[40]; Figge and Piater[41 42 43 44 45 46]; Figge and Schoene[47]; Piater and Figge[48]; vom Bruck, Figge, Piater and Wolf[49]; vom Bruck, Figge and Wolf[50]. These papers have also reported studies on whether defined synthetic triglycerides, free of unsaponifiable matter and of analytically interfering constituents, or other liquids would better simulate the extraction effect of fatty foodstuffs than the simulants proposed hitherto.

In order to simulate the migration of additives under conditions of use by
model tests in a reasonably short time, Figge[51] studied the influence of
temperature and time on the migration of additives. His investigations led
to the development of a simulant which is generally suitable for edible oils
and fatty foodstuffs (Figge et al[46]).

Figge[51] is of the opinion that the determination of amounts of extracted or
migrated additives in the parts per million range or lower can only be
carried out with the necessary accuracy by means of the radiotracer technique
(Figge and Piater[41] [45]; Figge and Schoene[47]; vom Bruck et al[50]). He
synthesized four representative plastics-processing additives with a
[14]C-label, as shown below. These were an organotin stabilizer (Figge[52])
a phenolic antioxidant (Figge[53]) and two lubricants.

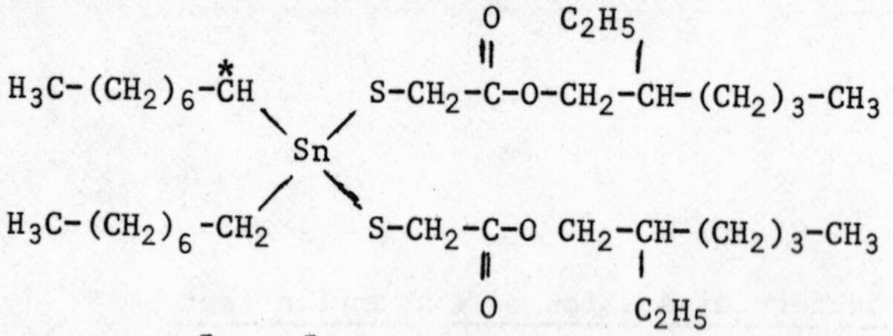

$$H_3C-(CH_2)_6-\overset{*}{C}H$$
$$H_3C-(CH_2)_6-CH_2$$
$$Sn$$

$$\overset{O}{\underset{\|}{}}\quad\overset{C_2H_5}{\underset{|}{}}$$
$$S-CH_2-C-O-CH_2-CH-(CH_2)_3-CH_3$$

$$S-CH_2-C-O\quad CH_2-CH-(CH_2)_3-CH_3$$
$$\underset{\|}{}\qquad\underset{|}{}$$
$$O\qquad C_2H_5$$

Di-n-octyl[1-^{14}C]-tin-2-ethyl-n-hexyl dithioglycollate
(Advastab (now Irgastab) 17 MOK-[^{14}C])

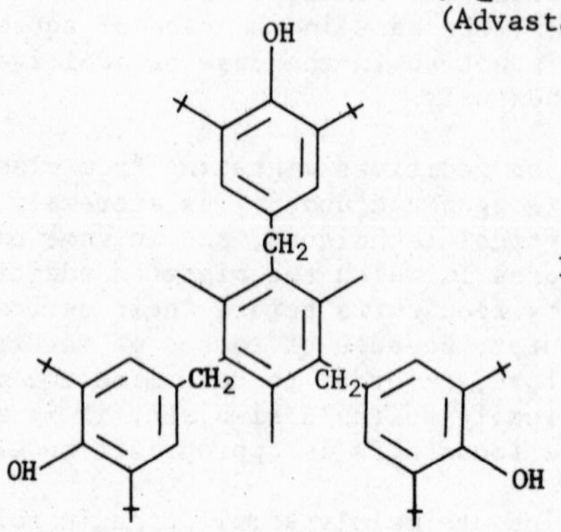

1,3,5-Trimethyl-2,4,6-tris-(3,5-di-tert-
butyl-4-hydroxybenzyl [^{14}C] benzene
(Ionox 330-[^{14}C])

$$H_3C-(CH_2)_{16}-\overset{*}{\underset{\|}{C}}-O-CH_2-(CH_2)_2-CH_3$$
$$O$$

n-Butyl stearate [1-^{14}C]

$$H_3C-CH_2)_{16}-\overset{*}{\underset{\|}{C}}-NH_2$$
$$O$$

Stearic acid[1-^{14}C] amide

The plastics used in the investigation by Figge[51] were polyvinyl chloride (PVC)
polystyrene (PS) and high-density polyethylene (HD-PE), materials widely used
in packaging fatty foodstuffs. In some experiments, low-density polyethylene
(LD-PE) was also included. The plastics were admixed with radioactive and
inactive additives to yield the plastics compositions described in Table 9.
For each type of plastics, two mixtures of the same percentage composition
were prepared, differing only in the additive carrying the radioactive labelling.
Using a laboratory extruder, the mixtures were then extruded to test films,
the physical and chemical properties of which corresponded to those of films

made on a factory scale. A comparative determination of the amounts of additive
migrating into different contact media is only possible if the radioactive
indicators are uniformly distributed over the area and mass of the test films.
Therefore, Figge[51] checked the evenness of their distribution
in longitudinal and transverse directions in the films by direct
continuous measuring methods as well as by autoradiography. In the film mass,
the homogeneity was checked by liquid scintillation measurements (Figge and
Schoene[47]).

The comparative extraction and migration tests were carried out under two
different sets of experimental conditions:

(a) All-sided extraction of film chips by edible oils or fat simulants for
    5 hours at 65°C, in accordance with the recommendations (Franck[34]) given
    by the Bundesgesundheitsamt (extraction or short-term tests).

(b) Migration during one-sided contact between the test film and the edible
    oil or fat simulant for 30 or 60 days at 20°C and 65% relative humidity,
    corresponding to the usual storage of edible oils in plastics containers
    (one-sided migration or long-term tests).

The fat simulants used were n-heptane (Food and Drug Administration[3]; Italian
Ministry of Health[33]), diethyl ether (Franck[34]), paraffin oil (British
Plastics Federation[1]) and others which have been proposed by different
authorities. In addition triglycerides and triglyceride mixtures were
included in the tests. The migration and extraction properties of these
simulants we r e compared with those of olive oil, sunflowerseed oil, coconut
oil, butter, Biskin*and SB margarine*. (*both manufactured by Margarine-
Union GmbH, Hamburg; SB margarine is a water/oil emulsion, thus the oil is
the outer phase).

For the migration tests with solid and liquid contact media different migration
cells were used (Figge and Piater[41] [45]) (Figs. 19 and 20). With these cells
it proved possible to effect a one-sided contact between the test film and
the fat or simulant, under constant contact conditions. The migration cells
consisted substantially of two outer rings of similar shape and equal size
and an inner ring. When the migration cells were filled, care was taken
that no air bubbles remained between the test film and the fat or simulant.
In the case of cells of the type shown in Fig.19, the inner rings were
equipped with sealable bore holes to allow for samples to be taken during
the test period.

Details of the method and the evaluation of the tests are discussed later
in this Chapter (Figge and Piater[41] [43] [45])

Figge[51] found that the interactions between different edible oils and a plastics
simulent extraction liquid were so similar that it seemed possible to develop a
standard fat simulant (Table 10). The amounts of additive migrating from a
given plastics into the four edible oils investigated differed at most by a
factor of about 3.5. If we consider the safety factors of 100 or 500 or more,
by which the toxicological no-effect levels determined in animals are usually
reduced, then this difference is not critical.

TABLE 9

Identification of Radioactive Test Films

Plastics mixtures			Test films		
Type	Components	Levels (% w/w)	Designation	^{14}C-labelled additive	Specific radioactivity (nC/g)
LD-DE	LD-PE Lupolen 1800 H	98.8			
	Ionox 330	1.0	LD-PE-Io	Ionox 330–[^{14}C]*	586
	Stearic acid amide	0.2	LD-PE-Sa	Stearic acid [1–^{14}C]amide	566
HD-PE	HD-PE Lupolen 5261 Z	98.8			
	Ionox 330	1.0	HD-PE-Io	Ionox 330–[^{14}C]*	525
	Stearic acid amide	0.2	HD-PE-Sa	Stearic acid [1–^{14}C]amide	525
PVC	PVC Solvic 229	97.0			
	Advastab 17 MOK	1.5	PVC-Sn	Advastab 17 MOK– [^{14}C]†	508
	Stenol 1618‡	0.6			
	Ionox 330	0.5	PVC-Io	Ionox 330– [^{14}C]*	487
	Loxiol G10§	0.4			
PS	PS BASF KR 2570/2	97.5			
	Ionox 330	2.0	PS-Io	Ionox 330– [^{14}C]*	458
	n-Butyl stearate	0.5	PS-Sb	n-Butyl stearate[1–^{14}C]	521

1,3,5-Trimethyl-2,4,6-tris-(3,5-di-tert-butyl-4-hydroxybenzyl [^{14}C])-benzene.

†Di-n-octyl [1–^{14}C]-tin-2-ethyl-n-hexyldithioglycollate.

‡Cetyl-stearyl alcohol, Deutsche Hydrierwerke GmbH, Düsseldorf.

§Ricinoleic acid monoglyceride, O. Neynaber, Loxstedt, BRD.

LD-PE:low density polyethylene; HD-PE:high density polyethylene; PS:polystyrene; PVC:polyvinyl chloride

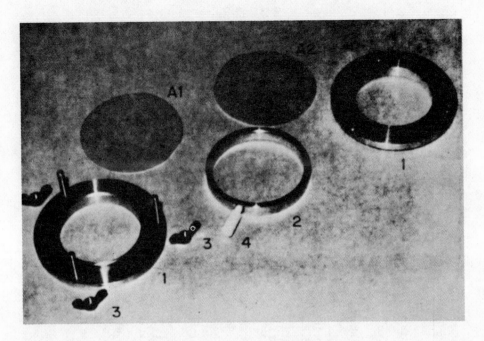

FIG.19   Migration cell from one-sided contact of polymer films with liquids,
          showing
          (a) Separate parts (1,outer rings, outer diameter 92mm); 2,inner ring
              (inner diameter 59mm); 3,bolt screws with wing nuts; 4,Teflon plug;
              A1 and A2, test film) and

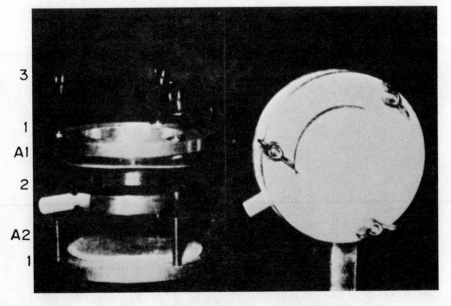

(b) the arrangements of the parts and the assembled cell.

TABLE 10

Transfer of Additives from Plastics Films into Edible Oils

Test film (and Additive)		Migration* of additive (%) into				Extractant† of additive (%) by		
No.	Designation	Sunflower-seed oil	Olive Oil	Biskin	SB margarine	Sunflower-seed oil	Olive Oil	Biskin
1	LD-PE-Io (Ionox 330)	36.8	35.6	–	–	88.8	91.8	93.4
3	HD-PE-Io (Ionox 330)	0.181	0.245	0.166	0.177	2.63	2.60	2.78
4	HD-PE-Sa (stearic acid amide)	2.09	1.67	3.80	3.90	46.8	55.8	57.0
5	PVC-Io (Ionox 330)	0.024	0.018	0.011	0.012	0.010	0.011	0.010
6	PVC-Sn (Advastab 17 MOK)	0.019	0.015	0.008	0.006	0.008	0.011	0.042
7	PS-Io (Ionox 330)	3.02	2.85	0.885	1.10	1.24	0.767	0.652
8	PS-Sb (n-butyl stearate)	4.58	4.53	1.98	3.46	1.79	1.16	0.960

LD-PE:low density polyethylene; HD-PE:high density polyethylene; PS:polystyrene; PVC:polyvinyl chloride

* One-sided contact for 60 days at 20°C and 65% relative humidity. (Migration defined as transfer of additives under storage conditions, i.e. at or below 20°C and 65% relative humidity)

† All-round contact for 5 hours at 65°C (Extraction defined as elimination of additives from a packaging material, under extreme experimental conditions, e.g. at 65°C or at boiling heat frequently with low boiling liquids.)

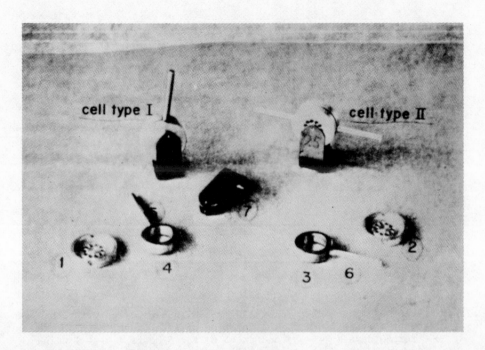

FIG.20 Migration cell for one-sided contact between test film and solid fat
        showing the separate parts (1) and (2), aluminium cover plates (outer
        diameter 22mm; (3) and (4) stainless steel rings (inner diameter 12mm;
        (5) metal handles; (6) glass suction tubes; (7) stainless steel clamp),
        the arrangement of these parts and the assembled cell of types I and II.

As was to be expected, the amounts of a given additive migrating from
different plastics into any one edible oil differed widely. The amounts of
Ionox 330 migrating into olive oil from PVC, low and high density polyethylene
and polystyrene, for instance, were in the proportions 1:14:160:2000 (Table
10). (The considerable migration of the large Ionox 330 molecule from low
density polyethylene at 20^{8}C confirms that this polymer cannot be
recommended for packaging fatty foods.) The migration of different
additives from the same plastics into a given edible oil also varied widely.
Thus, the migration of the lubricant, stearic acid amide, from high density
polyethylene was about 11-23 times higher than that of the antioxidant,
Ionox 330 (Table 10).

Even under extraction conditions (i.e. at a higher test temperature), the
interactions between different edible oils and a given plastics material were
similar (Table 10). Further investigations showed this conformity to apply
also to fats with a higher amount of medium-chain fatty acids, such as
butter fat or coconut oil. Edible oils thus behave so similarly that any
one of them could serve as a standard fat simulant for all other oils and
fats. However, for laboratory work, substances are preferred that can
more easily by analysed, provided they are also appropriate fat simulants
under migration and extraction conditions and this lead Figge [51] to
investigate the possibility of developing a single standard fatty simulant
liquid for use in extraction tests.

Results with different organic solvents and synthetic triglycerides and triglyceride mixtures are shown in Figures 21 to 23.

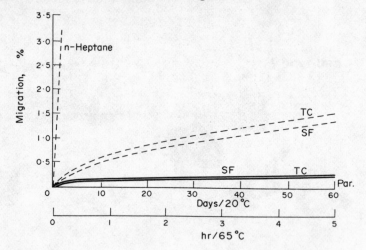

FIG.21 Migration of antioxidant Ionox 330 from high density polyethylene into different contact liquids as a function of time. Tests were carried out at 20°C for 60 days (-----) and at 65°C) for 5 hours (———) using sunflowerseed oil (SF), tricaprylin (TC) and paraffin oil (Par) and n-heptane.

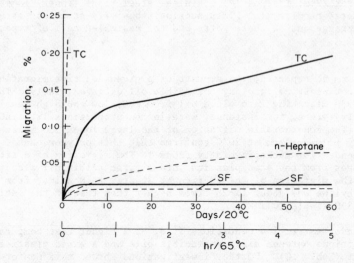

FIG.22 Migration of organotin stabilizer Avastab 17 MOK from PVC into different contact liquids as a function of time. Tests were carried out at 20°C for 60 days (------) and at 65°C for 5 hours (———) using sunflowerseed oil (SF), tricaprylin (TC) and n-heptane.

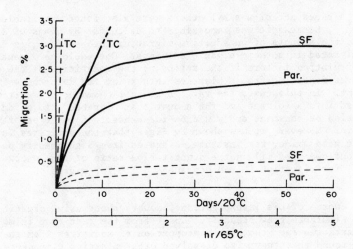

FIG.23 Migration of antioxidant Ionox 330 from polystyrene into different contact
        liquids as a function of time. Tests were carried out at 20°C for 60
        days (- - - -) and at 65°C for 5 hours (———) using sunflowerseed oil (SF),
        tricaprylin (TC) and n-heptane.

The synthetic triglyceride, tricaprylin, has been proposed by the French
authorities (Ministre de la Santé Publique[54] ,(1963). It is an excellent
fat simulant for the assessment of high density polyethylene packages. The
course of the migration with time of the phenolic antioxidant Ionox 330,
from high density polyethylene into tricaprylin (Fig.21) was in good
agreement with that into sunflowerseed oil. This conformity between
sunflowerseed oil and tricaprylin was also observed under extraction
conditions, at 65°C. However, tricaprylin is not a suitable fat simulant
for the assessment of PVC packages. Although the migration of the organotin
stabilizer from PCV into tricaprylin practically ceased after 60 days, it was
by that time about ten times higher than that obtained with sunflowerseed
oil (Fig.22). At 65°C tricaprylin causes so much swelling of PVC that
after 5 hours the degree of extraction is 250 times higher than that obtained
with sunflowerseed oil. The migration and extraction values of the
antioxidant, Ionox 330, from polystyrene (Fig.23) into tricaprylin are also
unrealistically high. These results show clearly that the medium-chain
triglyceride, tricaprylin, cannot be used as a standard fat simulant for
all types of plastic.

Figge[51] came to similar conclusions for the other fat simulants suggested
Although n-heptane, which has been proposed by authorities in the U S A
(Food and Drug Administration[3]) and Italy (Italian Ministry of Health[33])
could be used for PVC under extraction conditions (Fig.22) it extracted
more than 50% of the antioxidant, Ionox 330, from high density polyethylene
within 5 hours at 65°C (Fig.21). With paraffin oil, proposed by the
British Plastics Federation , the migration values for Ionox 330 from
polystyrene after 30 days at 20°C were similar to those obtained with
sunflowerseed oil. However, in contrast to sunflowerseed oil, paraffin oil
did not absorb measurable amounts of antioxidant from high density
polyethylene under migration conditions (Fig.21). Diethyl ether gave
extremely high extraction values compared to sunflowerseed oil in all the
additive/plastics combinations tested. Therefore, it must also be rejected
as a fat simulant.

Higher alkanes and di-n-alkyl ethers were also found unsuitable (Figge and
Piater[46]), because it was impossible to calculate by means of a few correlation
factors the amounts of an additive migrating into edible oils from the amounts
that migrated into these organic solvents. One could only manage with a
few correlation factors if the ratios of the quantities of the different
additives migrating from a plastics into a fat and into the solvent were
constant. In this case, the ratio between the amount of additive that
migrated into a solvent and the amount that migrated into an edible oil
would also be constant and would be independent of the type of plastics and
additive. However, it was shown by Figge that the additives Ionox 330 and
stearic acid amide, for instance, migrated from high density polyethylene
into sunflowerseed oil in the quantitative ratio of 1:8, whereas this ratio
was 1:1 for migration into n-heptane and 1:6 for migration into di-n-butyl
ether.

In the course of his investigations, doubts about using organic solvents
as fat simulants grew steadily. Apart from the fact that in most cases
they extracted far too high a proportion of additives from the plastics,
it was found that they also dissolved other plastics components. n-Heptane,
for instance, extracted more than 50% of plastics components from high
density polyethylene while n-heptane, diethyl ether or methanol extracted
between 70 and 99% from PVC and polystyrene. In the case of PVC, the
components concerned could possibly have been the added lubricants, but with
high density polyethylene and polystyrene they could only have consisted
of polymeric constituents.

The factor $F_M = \dfrac{\text{ppm dry matter of solvent extract}}{\text{ppm } {}^{14}\text{C-labelled additive in sunflowerseed oil}}$

differed from plastics to plastics and from extractant to extractant, but
the total extract as determined gravimetrically was always considerably
higher than the amount of ^{14}C-labelled additives that migrated into
sunflowerseed oil (Piater and Figge[48]).

The results show that there is no utilizable relation between the degree of
total extraction with organic solvents and the amounts of an additive or
the total amount of material migrating from plastics into the edible oil.
The total extract with organic solvents can only indicate the analytical
efforts required for the determination of certain additives, the daily
consumption of which in food should be restricted. Moreover, total
extracts of different batches of the same plastics enable the batches to be
checked for identical behaviour.

Thus, there is no doubt that an organic solvent, such as n-heptane or
diethyl ether, differing completely in chemical structure from an edible
oil and showing different properties of interaction towards the plastics
material, can never be a true fat simulant.

In all, Figge[51] studied as extractant liquids, organic solvents and
tricaprylin (Figures 21 to 23), triacetin, MCT (a mixture of medium-chain
triglycerides), tricaprin and HCFA-T (a mixture of hydrogenated cyclic
fatty acid triglycerides). In view of his own findings, discussed above,
and the fact that tricaprylin, MCT and tricaprin seriously attacked certain
types of plastics thereby causing smelling (vom Bruck[49]), Figge[51] then
concentrated his efforts on the development of a suitable fat simulant of
the synthetic triglyceride type.

Initially, he compared the transfer of individual C-labelled additives from different plastics into synthetic triglycerides or edible oils under migration conditions with that under extraction conditions.

It was a common feature of the plastics materials investigated that additive migration into glycerides was markedly reduced at low temperatures. This property is decisive for the utilization of plastics as packaging materials for fatty foods, particularly if they are to remain in cold-store to assist keeping.

Table 11 shows that where

$$Q = \frac{\text{final value of migration of extraction of additive in column 3}}{\text{final value of migration or extraction of Ionox 330}}$$

the ratio Q, for the migration values is nearly equal to that for the extraction values. This means that, with increasing test temperature, the additives of a plastics material migrate increasingly but at a constant quantitative ratio into synthetic triglycerides and edible oils. Moreover, the Q values for synthetic triglycerides are in good agreement with those for edible oils. Consequently, with the help of correlation factors still to be determined, it is possible to calculate the natural migration of plastics additives into edible oils from the corresponding extraction values with synthetic triglycerides. In view of these results, further investigations on the development of a standard triglyceride could be confined to either extraction or migration tests.

TABLE 11

Comparison of the Transfer of Additives from Different Polymers into Synthetic Triglycerides or Edible Oils at 20°C in 60 days and at 65°C in 5 hrs

Test film			Migration or extraction temp. ($^{\circ}$C)	Q† for contact medium	
Type	No.*			Synthetic triglyceride‡	Edible Oils§
HD-PE	3+4	Stearic acid amide	20	16	21
			65	20	20
PVC	5+6	Advastab 17 MOK	20	0.9	0.8
			65	1.2	0.8
PS	7+8	n-Butyl stearate	20	1.6	1.8
			65	1.9	1.5

HD-PE:high density polyethylene; PS:polystyrene; PVC:polyvinylchloride
*See Table 10

$$†Q = \frac{\text{final value of migration or extraction of additive in column 3}}{\text{final value of migration or extraction of Ionox 330}}$$

Q was calculated for all combinations of the test film and synthetic triglyceride or edible oil, and the mean value was calculated.

Footnote to Table 11 continued
‡ Tricaprylin, MCT and tricaprin.
§ Olive oil, sunflowerseed oil, Biskin, coconut oil and margarine.

An essential factor in the selection of a suitable triglyceride or triglyceride
mixture was the finding that triglycerides with medium-long straight-chain acyl
residues, such as tricaprylin, yield particularly high extraction and migration
rates compared with edible oils. The dependence of the amounts of additives that
migrated from different plastics films into triglycerides on the length of the
acyl residues has been systematically determined (Figge[51]). The amounts of
additives extracted by triglycerides from high density polyethylene, PVC or
polystyrene passed through distinct maxima when plotted against the length of the
acyl residue, as demonstrated by the curves in Figure 24.

Whereas the amounts of additives extracted from high density polyethylene increase
only slowly with increasing length of the acyl residue, pass through broad maxima
at 5-10 acyl C-atoms and then drop still more slowly, the curves for PVC and
polystyrene show very sharp maxima in the range of 3-5 acyl C-atoms: from trilaurin
or trimyristin onwards they remain practically constant. The height of the peak,
i.e. the maximally extracted amount of additive, differs widely from one plastics
to any other. With 2 hours at 65°C, the maximum removal of the antioxidant
Ionox 330, for instance, is 2% from high density polyethylene by tripelargonin,
57% from PVC by tributyrin and 100% from polystyrene by compounds between tripropin
and tricaprin.

As the migration values depend on the chain length of the acyl residues, it seems
reasonable to use a mixture of synthetic triglycerides as a fat simulant.
Figge[31] chose a blend with a fatty acid composition similar to the very strongly
extracting coconut oil.

In order to ensure that simple methods could be used for the analysis of additives
in the fat simulant, it was found necessary for the standard triglyceride mixture
to have the following chemical constants; unsaponifiable matter <0.4%; acid value
iodine value <1 (acid value and iodine value determined by respectively,
DGF-Einheitsmethode C-III 1b (53), C-V2 (57) and C-V 11d (53), (Standard Methods
of Analysing Fats and Oils), Deutsche Forschungsgemeinschaft, Wissenschaftliche
Verlagsgesellschaft mbH, Stuttgart). It also needed to be free of nitrogen and
phosphorous-containing substances, and to have a total content of mono- and
diglycerides not exceeding 2.5%, while fatty acids were required to be saturated
and randomly distributed among all the triglycerides of the mixture.

Again, for analytical convenience, it is desirable that the limit of optical
transmission (optical transmission is that wavelength at which the extinction of
the undiluted substance (1 cm cuvette; reference cuvette: water) approximates
the value 1, which corresponds to an optical transmission of 10%), of the
standard triglyceride mixtures should lie below 330 nm. This would, for
instance, be important for the direct ultraviolet spectroscopic determination
of migrated additives in the simulant.

Figge[51] [40] developed a suitable method for the synthesis of a standard triglyceride
mixture which meets the above requirements.

A mixture of synthetic fatty acids was calculated from literature data on the
fatty acid composition of coconut oil. Apart from 50% (w/w) lauric acid, the
mixture contained 20.5% lower and 29.5% higher fatty acids. It was esterified
with glycerol without using a catalyst.

The fatty acid composition of the synthetic product agrees well with the mean
chain-length distribution of coconut oil. The triglyceride distribution of the

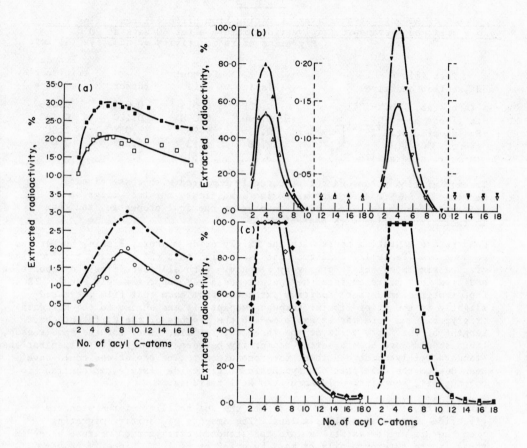

FIG.24 Dependence of the amount of radioactivity or additive extracted on the
chain-length of the acyl residue in triglycerides. Levels of extraction
were determined for:

(a) Stearamide (□) and Ionox 330 (0,0) from high density polyethylene,

(b) Avastab 17 MOK (▽) and Ionox 330 (△) from PVC and

(c) n-butyl stearate (□) and Ionox 330 (◇) from polystyrene after
    2 hours (open symbols) and 5 hours (solid symbols) at 65°C.

standard triglyceride mixture also corresponds to the mean triglyceride
distribution of coconut oil. Some of the analytical constants of the standard
triglyceride mixture are superior to those specified above. Thus, the product
contains only 0.1% unsaponifiable matter instead of 0.4%, diglycerides amounts
to only 1.3% compared to 2.5%. With these properties, the synthetic triglyceride
mixture shows the hoped-for analytical advantages over coconut oil.

The synthetic mixture does not contain impurities which could interfere with
the conventional analytical determination of migrated additives. Moreover,
it is very stable because of its saturated acyl residues (no autoxidation) and
it can be prepared in constant quality.

TABLE 12

Comparison of amounts of additives migrating from different test films into edible oils and a standard triglyceride mixture after 60 days at 20°C

Migration of radioactivity or additive (%) into

Test film (and labelled additive)	Biskin	Coconut Oil	Butter	Standard triglyceride mixture
PVC-Sn (Advastab 17 MOK-^{14}C)	0.009	0.014	0.017	0.016
HD-PE-Io (Ionox 330-^{14}C)	0.090	0.098	0.120	0.140
HD-PE-Sa (stearic acid $[1-^{14}C]$-amide)	0.80	0.96	1.05	1.36
PS-Io (Ionox 330-^{14}C)	2.08	2.53	3.07	3.05
PS-Sb (n-butyl stearate $[1-^{14}C]$)	5.20	5.61	7.11	7.57

These migration values cannot be directly compared with those already mentioned. Due to different extrusion conditions, the test films used differed from those used earlier in physico-chemical properties and thus in their interaction with contact media.

Comparative migration tests with the triglyceride mixture, Biskin, butter and coconut oil (Table 12) confirmed the assumption that the standard triglyceride mixture simulates edible oils very closely. With all test films the amounts of additive that migrated into the contact media were approximately equal. The fact that the amounts of additive extracted from each test film increased slightly in the order Biskin, through coconut oil and butter to the standard triglyceride mixture may be explained on the grounds of the different chain lengths of the fatty acids of the three edible oils. But, for the same reason, there should have been a better conformity between the migration values for the standard triglyceride and those for coconut oil. The deviations could have been due to the fact that the synthetic triglyceride mixture, in contrast to coconut oil, contained only saturated acyl residues.

However, these deviations do not impair the suitabiility of the standard glyceride mixture as a fat simulant. The amounts of additive migrating from the different test films into the standard triglyceride mixture exceeded those in the reference oils at most by a factor of 1.8. Since, moreover the migration of additives from plastics into Biskin is in good conformity with that into margarine, olive and sunflowerseed oil (Table 10). Figge[51] is of the opinion that this synthetic standard triglyceride mixture represents an appropriate, generally applicable simulant for pure edible oils and fatty foodstuffs. It has been successfully used in model tests for the assessment of the physiological acceptability of plastics packaging materials, and is being produced on a pilot plant scale under the name 'Fat Simulant HB 307' with the following analytical certificate:

Composition

Fatty acid distribution

No. of C-atoms in fatty acid residue (GLC% peak area): 6(1.2±1); 8(8.0±1); 10(10.4±1); 12(50.0±1); 14(13.6±1); 16(7.6±1); 18(8.4±1); others (0.8±0.5)

Typical triglyceride distribution (values not guaranteed)

Total no. of C-atmos in fatty acid residue (GLC% peak area): 22(0.1); 24(0.3); 26(1.0); 28(2.3); 30(4.9); 32(10.9); 34(13.9); 36(21.1); 38(16.1); 40(11.7); 42(9.8); 44(4.4); 46(2.2); 48(1.1); 50(0.2)

Purity

Monoglyceride content determined enzymatically, 0.2%
Diglyceride content determined enzymatically, 1.8%

Unsaponfiable matter (DGF-Einheitsmethods C-III lb 53), 0.2%
Iodine value (Wijs- DGF-Einheitsmethods C-V 11d 53), 1
Acid value (DGF-Einheitsmethods C-V2 57), 0.1
Water content (Karl Fischer), 0.1%
Melting point (clear), 28±2°C

Typical absorption spectrum (sample path length d=1cm; reference, water at
   35°C;

Wave length (nm)	290	310	330	350	370	390	430	470	510
Transmittance (%)	2	15	37	64	80	88	95	97	98

At least 10% light transmittance (1cm cuvette; reference, water at 35°C) at
300±10nm.

Details of extraction test apparatus (Figge and Piater[41,43,45])

Figge and Piater[41] have discussed three methods for the determination and
simulation of the migration off[14]C-labelled plastics additives from test
films into edible oils or model liquids as a function of time:

1. Extraction of film chips on all sides for 5 hours at 65°C following up a
   method recommended by the German Federal Ministry of Health using the
   synthetic triglyceride mixture HB307, liquid paraffin, diethyl ether,
   n-heptane and methanol as extractant liquids.

2. Migration of additives from films on one side in contact with the contents
   packed.   The test covers 60 days at 20°C 65% r. h. in accordance with
   the conventional storage conditions of edible oils in plastics containers.

3. Migration of additives from films on both sides in contact with the
   contents packed.

The apparatus for studying the migration of additives from films on one
side with the extractant is illustrated in Figures 19 (liquids) 20 and 25
(solid fats) and for studying the migration of additives from films on both
sides in contact with the extractant in Figure 26.

For scintillation counting of the concentration of extracted labelled additive
in the fatty foodstuff simulant they used a Tri-carb scintillation spectrometer
Model 3314 (Packard Instrument Co. U.S.A.) employing a mixture of 4g 2, 5 -
diphenyloxazol and 0.3g 1, 4 bis-2-(4methyl-5-phenyloxazolyl)-benzol in
1 litre of Merck 8325 toluene as the scintillation liquid. The contact area
between plastic film and simulant liquid was varied between 28.25cm^2 and
67.93cm^2. In any particular series of tests the contact area of film and
the volume of the extraction cell was kept constant. Figge and Piater[41,55-61]
developed formulae for the calculation of the corrected time dependent migration
rates (%) from their radioactivity measurements on the extractant after
specified time intervals.

Figge and Piater[41,43,45] studied the rate of migration at 65°C for up to
5 hours of various ^{14}C-labelled additives (di-n-octyl [1-^{14}C]-tin-dithioglycollic
acid-2ethyl-n-hexylester(Avastab 17 MOK-^{14}C), 1,3,5,-trimethyl-2,4,6-tris
(3,5-di-tert. butyl.-4hydroxybenzyl[14]C)-benzene, (Ionox 330-^{14}C, stearic acid-
[-^{14}C] amide and n-butylstearate 1[14]C incorporated into rigid PVC,
polystyrene, and high and low density polyethylene sheet and chips into materials
including triacetin (Figure 27) tricaprylin (Figs 28, 29, 30) medium chain

triglycerides (Figure 31), hydrogenated cyclic fatty acid triglycerides
(Figure 32), olive oil (Figure 33), margarine (Figure 34), Biskin (Figures
35, 36), sunflowerseed oil (Figure 37), and coconut oil (Figure 38), also
diethyl ether (Figure 39), n-heptane and paraffin oil (Figure 40).

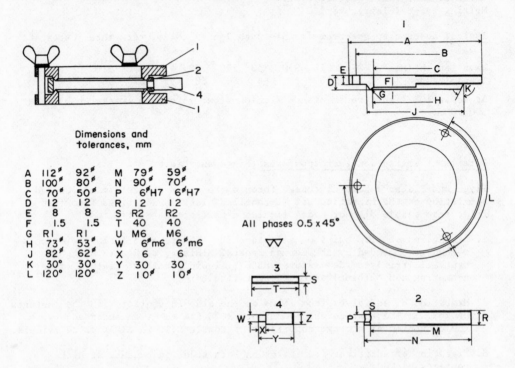

Dimensions and
tolerances, mm

A	112$^\phi$	92$^\phi$	M	79$^\phi$	59$^\phi$
B	100$^\phi$	80$^\phi$	N	90$^\phi$	70$^\phi$
C	70$^\phi$	50$^\phi$	P	6$^\phi$H7	6$^\phi$H7
D	12	12	R	12	12
E	8	8	S	R2	R2
F	1.5	1.5	T	40	40
G	R1	R1	U	M6	M6
H	73$^\phi$	53$^\phi$	W	6$^\phi$m6	6$^\phi$m6
J	82$^\phi$	62$^\phi$	X	6	6
K	30°	30°	Y	30	30
L	120°	120°	Z	10$^\phi$	10$^\phi$

All phases 0.5 x 45°

FIG.25 Migration cell for one-sided contact of plastic films with fats.

Extraction tests were performed at 20°C and 65°C. The effect of free fatty acids
present in some of the extractants was also ascertained (Figures 30-37).

The amounts of extracted additives were determined radiometrically.

Figge and Piater[45] have described the construction of special cells for
determining the rate of extraction and the depth of penetration of the
aforementioned labelled additives from one side of the plastic sheets (as opposed
to film) into solid fats during 60 days at 20°C at a relative humidity of 65%.
This apparatus is illustrated in Figures 26 and 41. The work is discussed
in further detail later on.

In order to increase the ratio of area of plastic film to volume of extractant
in·contact with the film in migration tests, Koch and Figge[62] experimented by
filling the cell with glass beads. Experiments with PVC films containing 5% or
20% of ^{14}C-labelled 2-ethyl-hexyl-phthalate showed that the migration of additive
into the fat simulant HB307 is not hindered by the very limited area of
contact (Table 13) between the plastics surface and the glass beads. The main
advantages of this method are its simplicity and the improved enrichment of
additives in the fat simulant which facilitates the determination of the specific
migration.

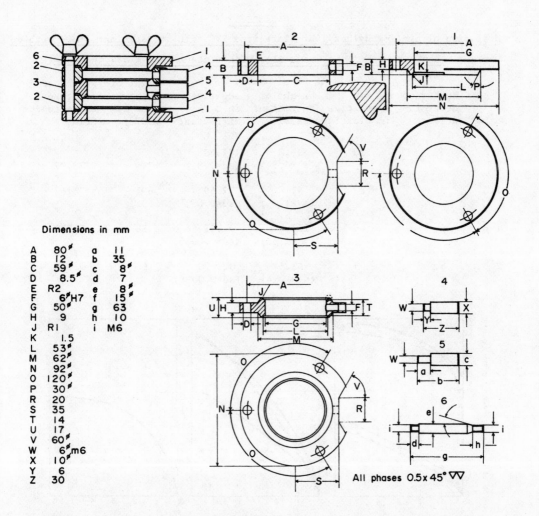

Dimensions in mm

A	80	a	11
B	12	b	35
C	59	c	8
D	8.5	d	7
E	R2	e	8
F	6 H7	f	15
G	50	g	63
H	9	h	10
J	R1	i	M6
K	1.5		
L	53		
M	62		
N	92		
O	120		
P	30		
R	20		
S	35		
T	14		
U	17		
V	60		
W	6 m6		
X	10		
Y	6		
Z	30		

All phases 0.5 x 45°

FIG.26 Migration cell for two-sided contact of plastic films with fats.

In more recent work Figge and Koch[63] confirm that organic liquids such as alkanes
and di-n-alkyl ethers are unsatisfactory for use as fat simulants and that a
synthetic analytically pure triglyceride mixture which has a fatty acid and
triglyceride distribution similar to that of coconut oil is a universally applicable
simulant for edible oils and fat containing foodstuffs. They studied the influence
of temperature on the migration of additives from PVC, high density polyethylene
and polystyrene into edible oils and into HB307. For edible fats and fatty
foodstuffs packed in plastics materials, the normal storage time prior to sale and
in the home is considered to be between 3 and 6 months at room temperature.
Van der Heide[64] has suggested an accelerated storage test of 10 days at 45°C for
the rapid determination of migration. Using different systems of plastics and
edible fats, he showed that under these conditions, the same additive transfer
occurred as during storage at 25°C for 6 months. These findings have been
confirmed by Waggon and others[65,66]. In his earlier investigations (Figge and
Piater[44,45]) Figge found that after 30 days at 20°C there is generally no longer

TABLE 13

Migration of di-(2-ethylhexylphthalate from PVC into fat simulant HB307 without contact with glass beads (1), with contact with glass beads (2)

Number	Number of determin- ations	% additive in plastic	Weight of extractant (HB307)	% of additive in extractant	Weight of additive found in HB307	Weight of additive extracted/dm^2 film
1 A	5	20	119.0 (s_m=0.54)	21.42 (sd=0.32)	1244	73.97
2 A	5	20	41.0 (s_m=1.01)	22.59 (sd=0.63)	3691	75.63
1 B	5	5	117.2 (s_m=1.56)	0.061 (sd=0.0036)	0.88	0.052
2 B	5	5	41.5 (s_m=1.14)	0.0670 (sd=0.0098)	2.80	0.058

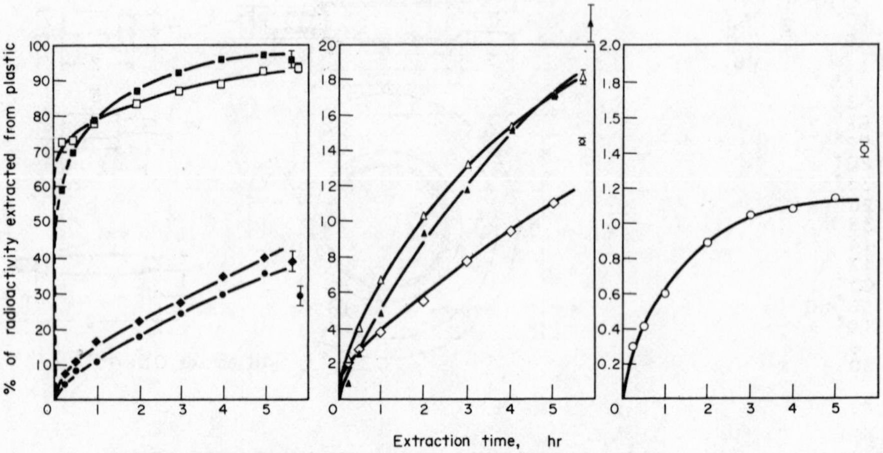

■ High density polyethylene-stearamide △ PVC-Ionox 330
□ High density polyethylene-Ionox 330 ▲ PVC-Avastab 17 MOK
♦ Polystyrene-n-butyl stearate ◇ Polystyrene-Ionox 330
● Low density polyethylene + stearamide ○ Low density polyethylene-Ionox 330

FIG. 27 Extraction curves, stearamide, Ionox 330, n-butyl stearate and Avastab 17 MOK from polyethylene, polystyrene and PVC into Triacetin at 65°C

a noticeable increase in the additive concentration either in edible fats or in simulant HB307. Consequently, storage tests at 20°C need not exceed 30 days duration and to shorten the test extraction temperatures of 40-50°C must be considered. In fact, as discussed below, Figge and Koch[63] found that, for all the polymer/additive combinations they investigated, additive migration into the fat simulant increased markedly above a test temperature of 50°C. The intensity of this increase and the temperature at which it became apparant was found to depend on the type of plastic material and the physico-chemical properties of additive. The amount of additive migrating is largely independent of the depth of the layer of HB307 (i.e. the ratio of contact area to amount of simulant), as studies with

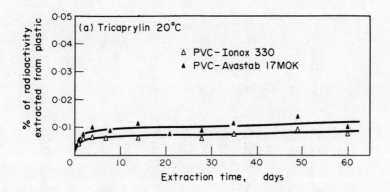

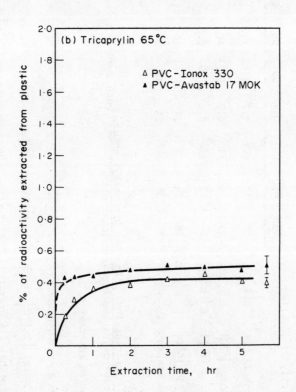

FIG.28   Extraction curves, Avastab 17 MOK and Ionox 330 from PVC into
         Tricaprylin:

    (a) at 20°C,
    (b) at 65°C.

simulant layers varying from 2.5 to 10mm have shown. As discussed below Figge
and Koch[63] used these results to define the conditions appropriate for the testing
of plastic films and containers intended for packaging edible oils and fatty
foodstuffs. Table 14 shows for different test films the ratios (R) between the
quantities of additive migrating into alkanes or di-n-alkyl ether and into
sunflower

TABLE 14

Comparison of the amounts of additive migrating from different test films into alkanes, di-n-alkyl ethers or sunflower oil in 60 days at 20°C and 65% relative humidity

R* for

Test film	Identity of labelled additive	Symmetric di-n-alkyl ethers†				n-Alkane†				Iso-octane
		C_8	C_{10}	C_{12}	C_{16}	C_7	C_9	C_{11}	C_{13}	
PVC	Irgastab 17 MOK-[14C]‡	30	17	6.1	1.2	2.1	1.3	0.8	0.6	0.6
HD-polyethylene	Ionox 330-[14C]§	23	15	11	6.0	55	40	31	21	16
	Stearic acid [1-14C] amide	17	13	11	8.2	7.0	6.2	5.8	5.6	4.3
Polystyrene	Ionox 330 [14C]	79	79	77	21	64	36	21	12	12
	n-Butyl stearate[1-14C]	35	35	34	21	34	34	34	28	22

*R = amount of additive migrating into alkane or di-n-alkyl ether, both amounts being expressed as a percentage / amount of additive migrating into sunflower oil

of the total amount in the test film.

† Total number of carbon atoms/molecule

‡ Heat stabilizer, di-n-octyl [1-14C] tin-bis-(2-ethylhexyl thioglycollate) (Figge52)

§ Antioxidant, 1,3,5-trimethyl-2,4,6-tris-(3,5-di-tert-butyl-4-hydroxybenzyl [14C])benzene (Figge53)

TABLE 15

Comparison of the amounts of additive migrating from different test films into edible fats and the fat simulant HB 307 during one-sided contact for 60 days at 20°C

Test film*	Identity & concn (% w/w) of labelled additive	Proportion (%) of radioactivity or additive migrating into				Ratio R† for		
		Biskin	Coconut Oil	Butter	HB 307	Biskin	Coconut Oil	Butter
Rigid PVC	Irgastab 17 MOK-$[^{14}C]$‡ (1.5)	0.009	0.014	0.017	0.016	1.8	1.1	1.0
HD polyethylene	Ionox 330-$[^{14}C]$§(1.0)	0.090	0.098	0.120	0.140	1.6	1.4	1.2
	Stearic acid$[1-^{14}C]$ amide (0.2)	0.80	0.96	1.05	1.36	1.7	1.4	1.3
Polystyrene	Ionox 330-$[^{14}C]$ (2.0)	2.08	2.53	3.07	3.05	1.5	1.2	1.0
	n-Butyl stearate $[1-^{14}C]$ (0.5)	5.20	5.61	7.11	7.57	1.5	1.4	1.1

* For performance of migration tests and composition of test films see Figge & Piater[41] and Figge & Schoene[47]

†R = $\dfrac{\text{amount of additive migrating into fat simulant HB 307}}{\text{amounts of additive migrating into Biskin, coconut oil or butter}}$

‡Di-n-octyl 1-$[C]$-tin-bis-(2-ethylhexylthioglycollate)(Figge[52])

§1,3,5-Trimethyl-2,4,6-tris-(3,5-tert-butyl-4-hydroxybenzyl$[^{14}C]$ benzene (Figge[53])

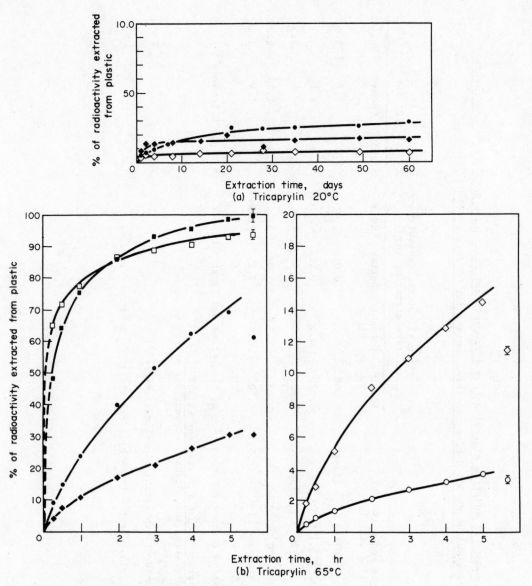

(a) Tricaprylin 20°C

(b) Tricaprylin 65°C

□ High density polyethylene–Ionox 330
■ High density polyethylene–stearamide
● Low density polyethylene–stearamide
◆ Polystyrene–n–butyl stearate
◇ Polystyrene–Ionox 330
○ Low density polyethylene–Ionox 330

FIG.29 Extraction curves, n-butyl stearate, Ionox 330, stearamide from polystyrene
and polyethylene into Tricaprylin:
(a) at 20°C,
(b) at 65°C

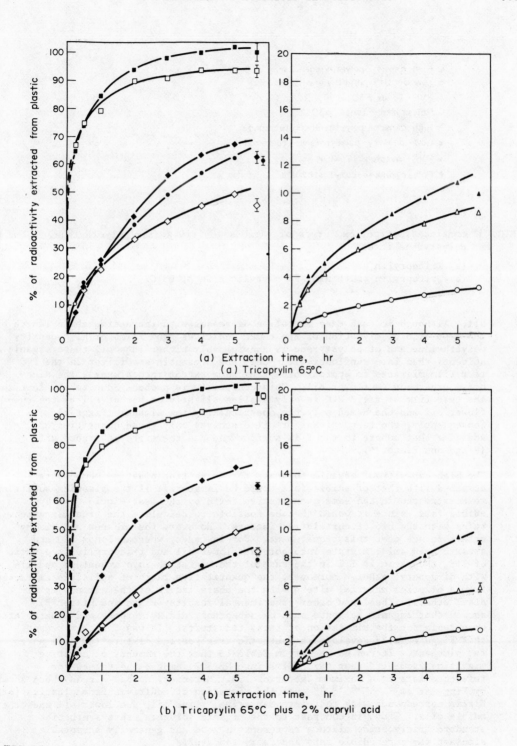

(a) Extraction time, hr
(a) Tricaprylin 65°C

(b) Extraction time, hr
(b) Tricaprylin 65°C plus 2% capryli acid

FIG. 30

□ High density polyethylene-Ionox 330
o Low density polyethylene-Ionox 330
Δ PVC-Ionox 330
◇ Polystyrene-Ionox 330
■ High density polyethylene-stearamide
• Low density polyethylene-stearamide
▲ PVC-Avastab 17 MOK
◆ Polystyrene-n-butyl stearate

FIG. 30 continued. Extraction curves of various additives from polyethylene, PVC and
    polystyrene into:

    (a) Tricaprylin,
    (b) Tricaprylin containing 2% caprylic acid at 65°C.

oil. Although in each case migration decreases with increasing chain length of
the test liquid, migration of the named additives from films of high density
polyethylene and of polystyrene is considerably higher into all these organic
solvents than into sunflower oil. Only the organotin stabilizer in the PVC
test film migrates to approximately the same extent into alkanes, the di-n-
octyl ether and sunflower oil. This conformity is probably due to the fact that
the test film of rigid PVC is only swollen slightly or not at all by the sunflower oil and the named solvents, particularly the alkanes (Figge[41]).
Consequently, the test solvent or oil dissolves only those quantities of
additive that adhere to the film surface and can therefore be washed off
(Figge and Piater[42]).

The high capacity of organic solvents for extracting plastics components
compared with that of edible fats would be immaterial if the plastics additives
were extracted in the same quantitative ratio by the test liquids and by
edible fats, since it would then be possible to calculate the true migration
rates with the aid of correlation factors. However, the alkanes and dialkyl
ethers do not meet this requirement. For instance, whereas Ionox 330 and
stearic acid amide migrate into both sunflower oil and tricaprylin in a ratio
of 1:8, the ratio is 1:1 in the case of the migration into n-heptane and 1:6
with di-n-butyl ether. Moreover, the quantitative ratio of additives extracted
from a plastics material alters with the chain length of the alkanes or dialkyl ethers. These and other experimental results (Figge and Piater[46])
showed that organic solvents such as n-heptane, dialkyl ethers and others, are
unsuitable for the simulation of fatty foddstuffs. It was for this reason
that Figge et al[40] developed a synthetic triglyceride mixture (HB 307) as a
fat simulant. It can be seen from Table 15 that the amounts of additive
migrating from different test films into HB 307, exceed the values for
reference fats by a maximum factor of 1.8. Moreover, as had already been shown
by Figge et al[39] [42-45] [48] [48] that the migration of additives from plastics into
Biskin corresponds with that into margarine, olive oil, sunflower oil and other
edible oils. Thus, in contrast to the organic solvents, this synthetic
standard triglyceride mixture represents a good and generally acceptable
simulant for pure edible fats and fatty foodstuffs.

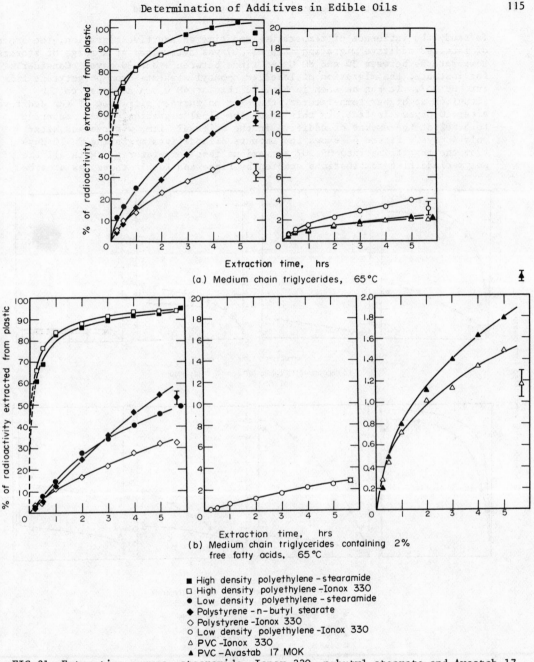

(a) Medium chain triglycerides, 65°C

Extraction time, hrs
(b) Medium chain triglycerides containing 2%
free fatty acids, 65°C

■ High density polyethylene – stearamide
□ High density polyethylene –Ionox 330
● Low density polyethylene – stearamide
◆ Polystyrene – n-butyl stearate
◇ Polystyrene –Ionox 330
○ Low density polyethylene –Ionox 330
△ PVC –Ionox 330
▲ PVC –Avastab 17 MOK

FIG.31 Extraction curves, stearamide, Ionox 330, n-butyl stearate and Avastab 17
MOK from polyethylene, polystyrene and PVC into:

(a) medium chain triglycerides,
(b) medium chain triglycerides containing 2% free fatty acid at 65°C.

6.2. Effect of extraction time and temperature on extractability of additives from plastics into fats

To study the influence of temperature and time an additive migration, the amount of labelled additive migrating into HB 307 was determined at a range of storage temperatures between 30 and 80°C and times between 1 and 30 days. Consider, for instance, the migration of labelled n-butyl stearate from polystyrene film into HB 307. It can be seen in Fig. 42 that at 40°C, in contrast to the situation at higher temperatures, there is no further migration of the additive after 10 days. In fact, in this case, the final migration value, amounting to 5.68% of the amount of additive in the original film, was reached after only 4 days. Figure 43 shows the amounts of additives migrating in 10 days from the test films into HB 307 at various test temperatures. With all the polymer/additive combinations studied by Figge and Koch[63] there was a marked

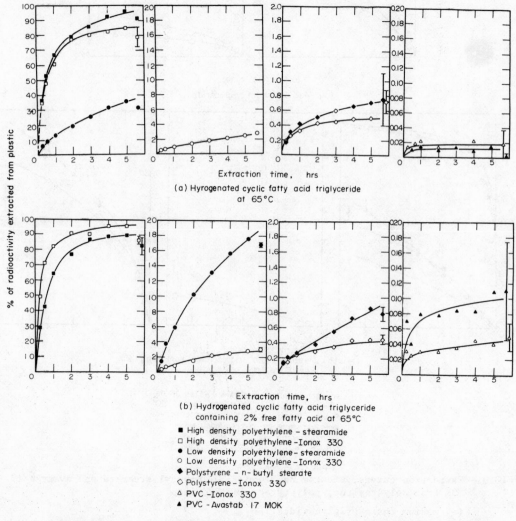

Extraction time, hrs
(a) Hyrogenated cyclic fatty acid triglyceride
at 65°C

Extraction time, hrs
(b) Hydrogenated cyclic fatty acid triglyceride
containing 2% free fatty acid at 65°C

■ High density polyethylene – stearamide
□ High density polyethylene –Ionox 330
● Low density polyethylene– stearamide
○ Low density polyethylene–Ionox 330
◆ Polystyrene – n–butyl stearate
◇ Polystyrene–Ionox 330
△ PVC –Ionox 330
▲ PVC –Avastab 17 MOK

FIG.32 Extraction curves, stearamide, Ionox 330, n-butyl stearate and Avastab 17 MOK from polyethylene into:

(a) hydrogenated cyclic fatty acid triglyceride,
(b) hydrogenated cyclic fatty acid triglyceride containing 2% free fatty acid at 65°C.

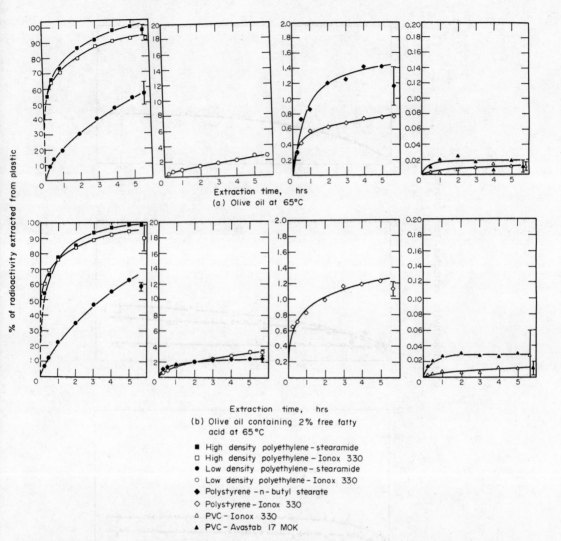

FIG.33   Extraction curves, stearamide, Ionox 330, n-butyl stearate and Avastab 17
MOK from polyethylene, polystyrene and PVC into:

(a) olive oil,
(b) olive oil containing 2% free fatty acids at 65°C.

increase in migration values above 50°C. The extent of this increase and the
point at which it began depended both on the type of plastics material and the
physico-chemical properties of the additive. Thus, while the migration of
Ionox 330 from either polystyrene or high density polyethylene showed a
marked increase only above 65°C, an increase in the migration of n-butyl
stearate from polystyrene and of stearic acid amide from high density
polyethylene was clearly observed at 50°C. Consequently, in order to simulate
migration under storage conditions, it is necessary to know the extent of this
increased migration and the temperature at which it begins to occur, since the
use of too high a test temperature could indicate an unrealistically high level

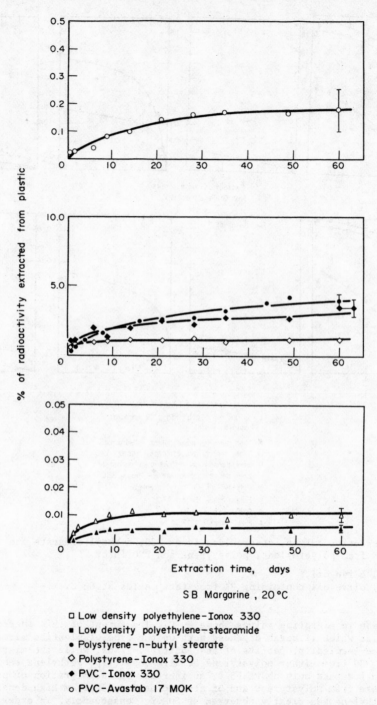

SB Margarine , 20°C

□ Low density polyethylene – Ionox 330
■ Low density polyethylene – stearamide
● Polystyrene – n–butyl stearate
◇ Polystyrene – Ionox 330
◆ PVC – Ionox 330
○ PVC – Avastab 17 MOK

FIG. 34 Extraction curves, Ionox 330, stearamide, n–butyl stearate and Avastab 17 MOK from low density polyethylene, polystyrene and PVC into SB Margarine at 20°C.

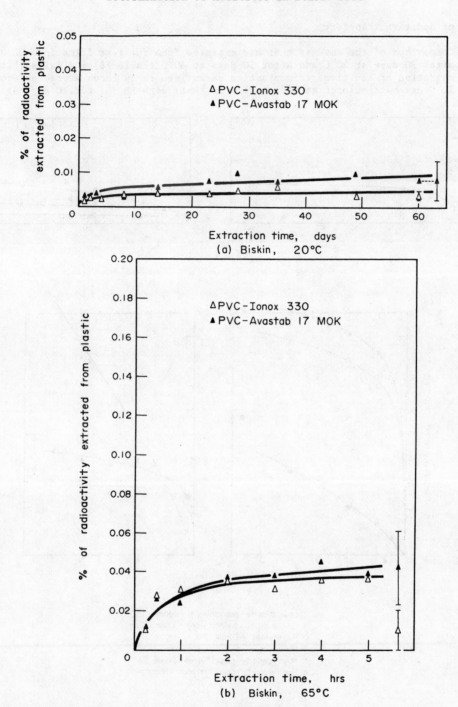

FIG.35 Extraction curves, Avastab 17 MOK and Ionox 330 from PVC into Biskin:

(a) at 20°C,
(b) at 65°C.

of additive transfer.

Comparison of the amounts that had migrated from the test films into HB 307 after 30 days at 20°C and after 10 days at 40°C (Table 16) indicates that the migration of additives from plastics packs into fatty foods stored at about 20°C can be simulated satisfactorily in tests with HB 307 for 10 days at 40°C.

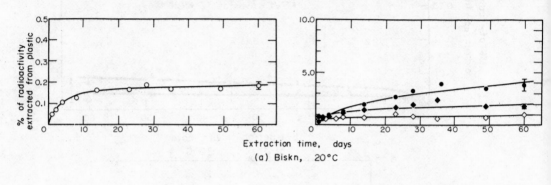

Extraction time, days

(a) Biskn, 20°C

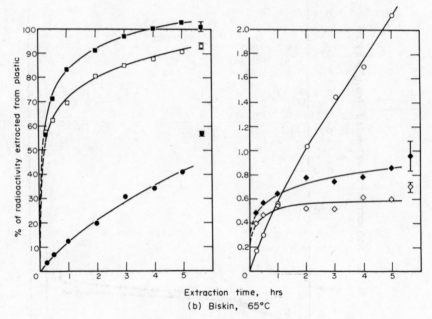

Extraction time, hrs

(b) Biskin, 65°C

○ Low density polyethylene – Ionox 330
● Low density polyethylene – stearamide
◇ Polystyrene – Ionox 330
◆ Polystyrene – n-butyl stearate
□ High density polyethylene – Ionox 330
■ High density polyethylene – stearamide

FIG.36 Extraction curves, Ionox 330, stearamide and n-butyl stearate from poly-
        ethylene and polystyrene into Biskin:

        (a) at 20°C,
        (b) at 65°C.

TABLE 16

Comparison of the amounts of additive migrating from different test
films into fat simulant HB 307 and coconut oil

		Migration of additive (%)		
		After 30 days at 20°C into		After 10 days at 40°C into
Test film	Labelled additive	Coconut Oil	HB 307	HB 307
PVC	Avastab 17 MOK-$[^{14}C]$	0.010	0.014	0.012
HD-polyethylene	Ionox 330-$[^{14}C]$	0.080	0.120	0.106
	Stearic acid$[1-^{14}C]$ amide	3.86	3.48	3.66
Polystyrene	Ionox 330-$[^{14}C]$	4.89	4.76	5.58
	n-Butyl stearate$[1-^{14}C]$	5.27	5.42	5.76

Figure 44 demonstrates that these facts also apply to rigid PVC films, which,
as already mentioned, are not swollen by fats at temperatures up to 60°C.
Two different rigid PVC films (Figge & Zeman[67]) containing the same stabilizer,
Avastab 17 MOK labelled with ^{14}C in the octyltin group were each found to
impart the same amounts of additive to HB 307 within 30 days at 20°C as within
10 days at 40°C. The amounts of radioactivity or stabilizer migrating from
the test film into the fat simulant were approximately equal under the
different test conditions and with both films the migration reached a constant
final value before test periods expired.

Figge and Koch[63] also studied the influence of the depth of the HB 307 layer
on the migration of additives from polymer films. To determine the extent
to which the ratio between the contact area and the volume of simulant (i.e.
the depth of the layer of HB 307 on the test material) affects the amount of
migration they designed migration cells of differing width but otherwise
identical construction. The basic design of these cells has been described
by Figge and Piater[41] and is shown in Fig. 45. With a constant area of
contact, the layers of simulant between pairs of test films fixed in the cells
parallel to each other were exactly 5, 10 or 20mm thick. These studies were
carried out with pressed films of PVC containing levels of di-(2ethyl-n-hexyl)
phthalate-$[^{14}C]$ between 4 and 25% (w/w) and extruded high density-polyethylene
film containing 1% (w/w) of the labelled antioxidant Ionox 330-$[^{14}C]$. Separate
determinations of plasticizer migration were carried out with each depth of
simulant studied and the mean amount of plasticizer was calculated in each
case. In addition, for each test film, the mean amounts of transferred
plasticizer and the coefficient of variation of the single results about the
mean were calculated thus giving a mean migration value independent of the
depth of the simulant layer.

The results of the study on the migration of plasticizer from PVC films into
different depths of HB 307 layers are given in Table 17. The extent of
migration of di-(2ethyl-n-hexyl) phthalate in 10 days at 40°C increased
marketly with increasing plasticizer content and the concentration of di-(2ethyl-
n-hexyl) phthalate in the simulant layers reached relatively high values.

TABLE 17

Migration of plasticizer from PVC test films into varying volumes of fat simulant HB 307

Content of di-(2ethyl-n-hexyl) phthalate (w/w)	PVC test film*								Migration of additive (%)‡ with a depth of simulant between two films of		
	Specific radioactivity										
	di(2ethyl-n-hexyl) 7,8¹⁴C phthalate		Film		Thickness		Weight		5mm	10mm	20mm
	μCi/g (n=10)	s%†	μCi/g (n=40)	s%†	μm (n=50)	s%†	mg/dm² (n=5)	s%† (n=5)			
4.0	104.21	1.17	4.139	2.71	222	7.3	2990.3	3.0	0.019(3.0)	0.017(2.1)	0.009(7.4)
6.0	70.92	1.11	4.225	1.24	224	11.2	2994.6	3.0	0.039(1.1)	0.039(2.7)	0.043(2.7)
9.0	34.90	1.06	3.162	1.96	218	11.8	3003.2	2.8	0.58(0.0)	0.51(1.9)	0.58(2.4)
12.0	34.90	1.06	4.155	1.57	220	7.0	2960.3	3.0	2.11(1.0)	2.13(1.4)	2.04(0.8)
16.0	34.90	1.06	5.823	2.07	210	5.5	2758.5	2.7	9.07(0.4)	8.73(0.8)	8.30(0.5)
20.0	34.90	1.06	6.878	2.24	216	5.6	2889.5	2.8	24.63(0.7)	22.51(0.9)	23.91(1.6)
25.0	34.90	1.06	8.617	1.58	213	4.8	2849.1	2.7	82.47(0.6)	79.76(0.4)	72.48(0.9)

* Composition: 95.0-74.0% (w/w) Vinoflex 503 (BASF, Ludwigshafen), 4.0-25.0% di-(2-ethyl-n-hexyl) [7,8-¹⁴C] phthalate), 0.5% Wachs E (Farbwerke Hoechst, Frankfurt/Main), 0.5% Stabilizer C (Farbenfabriken Bayer, Leverkusen).

† $s\% = \dfrac{\text{standard deviation}}{\text{mean value of n single values}} \times 100$

‡ Values in parentheses are the coefficients of variation (s%) of the single results about the mean of five determinations. Migration was determined after one-sided contact for 10 days at 40°C.

Nevertheless, the amounts of plasticiser AH migrating, for instances, from the PVC film containing 25% (w/w) of plasticizer into the different depths of fat simulant layers were approximately equal, and this similarity was even more marked with films containing lower levels of plasticizer. The curves in Fig.46 are the means of the 15 individual determinations of migration from each test film plotted as a function of the plasticizer content and the coefficient of variation of the single results about the mean. The narrow range of error confirms that the amounts of plasticizer migrating from the PVC test films into HB 307 are practically independent of the depth of the simulant layer. The amounts of the antioxidant, Ionox 330, that migrated from the high density-polyethylene film into HB 307 were 0.084, 0.082 and 0.069% with simulant layers of 5, 10 and 20mm, respectively.

Figge and Koch[63] consider, therefore, that a simulant layer of 5mm between two test films is sufficient for a migration test. This makes the quantitative

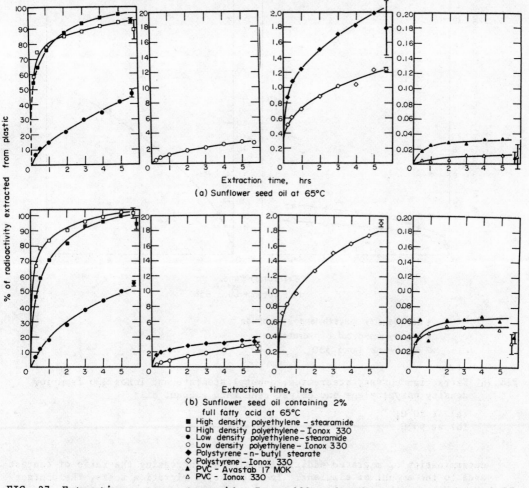

Extraction time, hrs

(a) Sunflower seed oil at 65°C

Extraction time, hrs

(b) Sunflower seed oil containing 2%
full fatty acid at 65°C

■ High density polyethylene – stearamide
□ High density polyethylene – Ionox 330
● Low density polyethylene – stearamide
○ Low density polyethylene – Ionox 330
◆ Polystyrene – n-butyl stearate
◇ Polystyrene – Ionox 330
▲ PVC – Avastab 17 MOK
△ PVC – Ionox 330

% of radioactivity extracted from plastic

FIG. 37 Extraction curves, stearamide, Ionox 330, n-butyl stearate and Avastab 17 MOK from polyethylene, polystyrene and PVC, into:

(a) sunflower seed oil,
(b) sunflower seed oil containing 2% free fatty acid at 65°C.

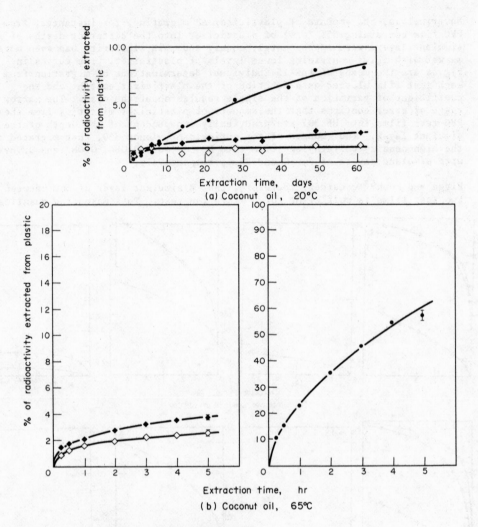

% of radioactivity extracted from plastic

(a) Coconut oil, 20°C

Extraction time, days

% of radioactivity extracted from plastic

Extraction time, hr

(b) Coconut oil, 65°C

• Low density polyethylene-stearamide
♦ Polystyrene-n-butyl stearate
◇ Polystyrene-Ionox 330

FIG.38 Extraction curves, stearamide, n-butyl stearate and Ionox 330 from low
density polyethylene and polystyrene into coconut oil:

(a) at 20°C,
(b) at 65°C.

determination of migrated additives easier by increasing the ratio of contact
area to the amount of simulant. In comparative migration tests, the contact
areas between the test film and test fat should be kept constant throughout
the study, since the amount of additive migrating in each case is proportional
to this area (Strodtz and Henry[59]). The design of the migration cell reflects
normal conditions of use, in that the test film is in one-sided contact with
the simulant. The final version of this migration cell provides a contact

area between the test film and the fat simulant of 2 × 50 cm and a simulant
layer 5mm in depth between the two circular films.

Figge and Koch[63] conclude that for test films used for packaging edible oils
and foodstuffs containing fats, it is appropriate to test migration into fat
simulant HB 307 (m.p. (clear) 29.3°C) in a migration cell providing a contact
area of 2 × 50cm , and a simulant layer 5mm in depth. After the required
amount of simulant has been placed in the cell, migration is tested either for
10 days at 40°C or under conditions actually encountered in practice. For
carrying out migration tests on plastics containers, the same fat simulant
and test conditions may be used, and when its volume and internal surface have
been determined, the container is filled with glass beads and the required
amount of simulant is placed in it. Analysis of the simulant follows either
type of contact and the resulting level of migrate in the simulant (µg/g) can
be converted to µg migrate/dm^2 contact area and thence to µg migrate/g foodstuff.

These workers stress that high temperatures encountered for limited periods
in practice (e.g. during pasteurization, sterilization or preparation of
foodstuffs in plastics packs) must be simulated by use of appropriate test

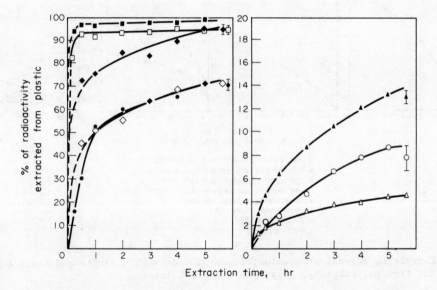

- ■ High density polyethylene-stearamide
- □ High density polyethylene-Ionox 330
- ◆ Polystyrene-n-butyl stearate
- ● Low density polyethylene-stearamide
- ◇ Polystyrene-Ionox 330
- ▲ PVC-Avastab 17 MOK
- ○ Low density polyethylene-Ionox 330
- △ PVC-Ionox 330

FIG. 39 Extraction curves, stearamide, Ionox 330, n-butyl stearate and Avastab 17
MOK from polyethylene, polystyrene and PVC into diethyl ether at 65°C.

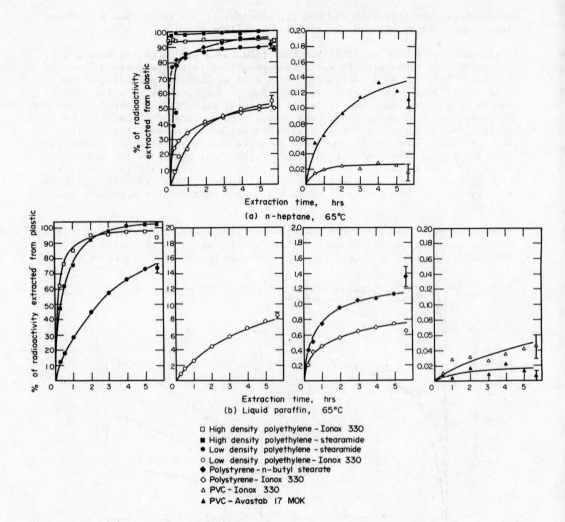

FIG.40   Extraction curves, stearamide, Ionox 330, n-butyl stearate and Avastab 17
         MOK from polyethylene, polystyrene and PVC into:

(a) n-heptane,
(b) liquid paraffin at 65°C.

temperatures and times. Moreoever, experimental films made only for test
purposes should be of the same thicknesses as the article that will actually
be used, since the thickness of the film has a definite influence on the
amount of additive migrating (Phillips and Marks[68 69]). The extent of
migration depends also on the physico-chemical properties of the test material,
including its density, surface quality and crystallinity. Test specimens,
both of films and plastics containers should therefore be made under standard
production conditions.

6.3. Determination of antioxidants and ultra-violet absorbers, heat stabilizers and plasticizers in fats

Although much of the published work in the determination of extracted polymer
additives in the synthetic triglyceride fat simulant HB 307 has been based on
radiochemical methods, using labelled additives, non-radiochemical methods
have been described. Koch and other workers have described methods, which are
based on alternative techniques such as visible and ultra-violet spectroscopy
and gas chromatography.

Koch[70] has described an ultra-violet spectroscopic method for the determination
of antioxidants, ultra-violet stabilizers and heat stabilizers and mixtures
thereof, the use of which are permitted by the German Bundesgesundheitampt
in the fat simulant HB 307. Figure 47 shows ultra-violet spectra of 10%,
20% and 50% solutions of HB 307 in chloroform, and a solution of 0.01% of the
2-ethylhexyl ester of thioglycollic acid and 10% HB 307 in chloroform. The
data in Table 18 shows the absorption maxima and lower detection limits for a
range of various types of polymer additives that can be determined in HB 307
with sensitivities ranging from 0.5 to 30ppm. In Fig.48 are shown calibration
curves obtained for solutions in chloroform and HB 307 of up to 10ppm of
2-(2'hydroxy-5'-methyl-phenyl)benzotriazole ultra-violet absorber, and thio-
ethylene-glycol-bis (β aminocrotonate) 2-phenylindole heat stabilizers.

Koch points out that for the determination of antioxidants in the parts per
million range it is advisable in this procedure to add thioglycollic acid
ester to protect the antioxidant against oxidation. The thioglycollic acid
ester should preferably be added to the fat simulant before the migration
test is started.

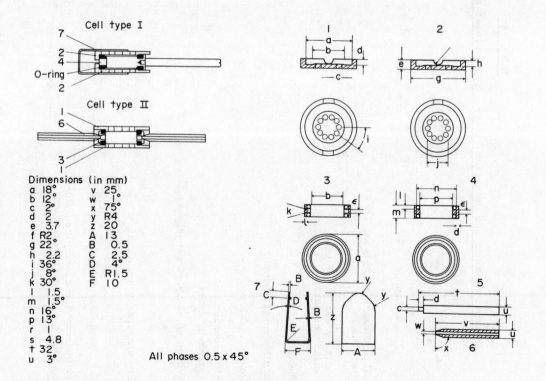

FIG.41 Migration cell for one-sided contact of plastic films with fats.

TABLE 18

Absorption maxima and detection limits. Ultra-violet spectroscopic determination of additives

No	Substance	Structure	Application	Type of polymer in which used	λ max nm	E 1% 1 cm	Lower detecn limit ppm
1	2-(2'-Hydroxy-5'methylphenyl)-benzotriazole		UV-Absorber	K,L,M,Q	297 337	602 710	1
2	Thiodiethylenglycol-bis(β-aminocrotonate)		Heat	M	275	1135	0,5
3	2-Phenylindole		Heat	M	309	1115	1
4	4,4'Dihydroxydiphenyl		Antioxidant	G,O	264	1170	0,5
5	Diphenylthiolurea		Heat	G,M,N	274	760	1
6	4,4'-Thio-bis-(6-tert-butylcresol)		Antioxidant	A,B,C,D,E,K,L,M	281	175	3
7	2,6-Di-tert,-butyl-4-methylphenol		Antioxidant	A,B,C,D,E,F,G,H,I,K,L,M,O,P	284	106,5	6
8	Tris-(nonylphenyl)-phosphite		Co-stabilizer	A,C,G,K,L,M	272	29	20
9	Dioctylphthalate		Plasticizer	K,L,M,R	275	28	20
10	S-(4-Hydroxy-3,5-dimethylbenzyl)-thioglycollic acid stearyl ester		Antioxidant	A,C,D	278	29	20

continued

TABLE 18 continued

No.	Name	Structure	Category			
11	3-Methyl-4-hydroxy-5-tert.-butyl-benzylmalonicaciddistearylester		Antioxidant A,C,D	278	19	30
12	Butandiol-bis-(β-aminocrotonate)		Heat M	275	1338	0,5
13	2,2'Methylene-bis-(4methyl-6-tert-butylphenol)		Antioxidant B,E,G,K,L,O,P	281	156	4
14	Bis-(3-cyclohexyl-5-methyl-2-hydroxyphenyl)-methane		Antioxidant B,E,G,K,L,O	283	138	4
15	2,2'-Methylene-bis-(4-ethyl-6-tert-butylphenol)		Antioxidant G	280	129	4
16	2,2-Bis-(4'-hydroxyphenyl)-propane		Antioxidant M,S	279	163	4
17	Bis- 3,3-bis-(4'-hydroxy-3'-tert butylphenyl)-butyricacid-glycolester		Antioxidant A,C,K,L	277 283	97,5 95,8	5
18	Tetrakis methylen-(3,5-di-tert.-butyl-4-hydroxyhydrocinnamate)-methane		Antioxidant A,B,C,D,F,M,P	276	63	8
19	β-(3,5-Di-tert-butyl-4-hydroxyphenyl)-propionicacid-n-octadecylester		Antioxidant A,B,C,D F,K,L,M	277	38	15
20	4,4'Butylidene-bis-(3-methyl-6-tert-butylphenol)		Antioxidant A,B,C,D, E,G,H,I, K,L,O,P.	237	117	5
21	Di-(2-hydroxy-5-tert-butylphenyl)-sulfide		Antioxidant E	291	227	3
22	1,3,5-Trimethyl-2,4,6-tris-(3',5'-di-tert-butyl-4'-hydroxybenzyl)-benzol		Antioxidant A,B,C,D,	278	91	6

TABLE 18 continued

No.	Name	Function	Polymer			
23	2+3-tert-Butyl-4-hydroxyanisole	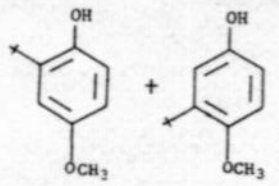 Antioxidant	A,B,C,D H,I,P	292	193	3
24	2-(2'-Hydroxy-3'-tert-butyl-5'-methylphenyl)-5-chlorbenzotriazole	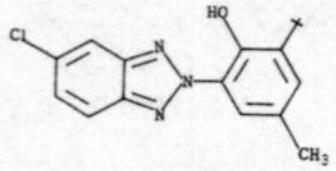 UV-Stabiliser	A,C,D	312 349	446 486	1
25	1,1,3-Tris-(2'methyl-4'-hydroxy-5'tert-butylphenyl)-butane	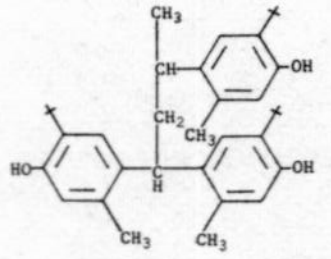 Antioxidant	C	267	133	4
26	2,5-Bis-5'-tert-butyl-benzoxazolyl-(2')-thiophen	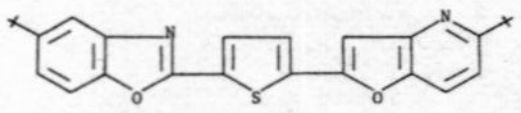 UV-Stabiliser	A,K,M	265 377	203 1153	0,5
27	2-Mercaptobenzothiazole	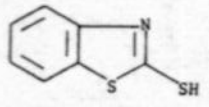 Vulcanising Agent	G	329	1720	0,4
28	Dibutylphthalate	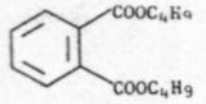 Plasticizer	M,R,T	274	44	12
29	Butylbenzylphthalate	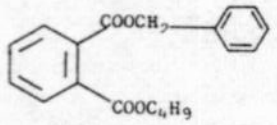 Plasticizer	M	274	43	12
30	Dicyclohexylphthalate	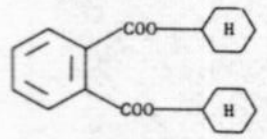 Plasticizer	M	274	39	13

A Polyethylene
B Ethylenecopolymer
C Polypropylene
C Polybutene (1)
E Polyisobutene
F Poly-4-methylpentene (1)
G Natur-und Synthesekautschuk
H Paraffin wax
I Microcrystalline wax
K Polystyrene
L Styrenecopolymers
M PVC
N Polychloroprene
O Dispersions
P Acetal
Q Polycarbonate
R Polyester-, Polyamide-, Polyurethane
S Silicones
T Homo- and copolymers

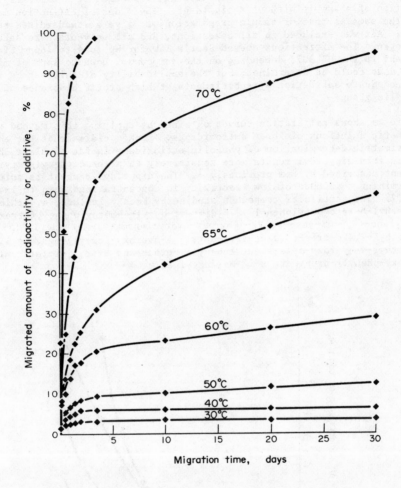

FIG.42 Migration of n-butyl stearate $[1-^{14}C]$ from polystyrene film into fat
        simulant HB 307 during periods of 1 to 30 days at temperatures between
        30 and 80°C.

Koch[71] [72] has also described visible colorimetric methods for the
determination of phenolic antioxidants and mercapto compounds in HB 307 in the
concentration range around 1 part per million. A method (Koch[71]) utilizing
diphenyl-picrylhydrazyl as the chromogenic reagent has been applied to the
determination of compounds such as 2,2' methylene-bis-(4-methyl-6-cyclo-
hexylphenol-1),2-ethyl-hexylthioglycollate,4,4'butylidene-bis-(-3-methyl-6-
tertiary-butylphenol-1) and 2,2'-methylene-bis-(-4-ethylene-6-tertiary-butyl
phenol-1). In this method, 2ml of an ethanolic solution (0.05 to 1mg per 100ml)
of an antioxidant was added to 5ml of a 50% solution of HB 307 in chloroform
or 1,2-dichloroethane in a stoppered test-tube.   Then 3ml of 0.0075%
ethanolic 2,2-diphenyl-1-picrylhydrazyl was added, and the stoppered tube was
heated for 30 or 60 minutes (according to the antioxidant) in a water bath at
60°C. The tube was cooled in water at 20°C, and, as soon as possible, the

extinction of the solution was measured at 517nm against a similarly prepared
solution of a sample without antioxidant. The order of extinction measurement
was the same as that of sample preparation, to give a standardised reaction
time. Air was excluded in all operations, and all solvents were saturated with
nitrogen. The extinctions obeyed Beer's law for up to 4 to 16ppm of antioxidant in the HB 307, depending on the compound. Down to 1ppm of many
compounds could be determined, but the applicability of this method is limited
by inadequate activation by substituents or high steric hindrance of the
phenolic group.

Figure 49 shows calibration curves obtained by applying this method to
synthetic solutions of three antioxidants. Koch[72] claims that for the direct
colorimetric determination of phenolic antioxidant in fat simulant HB 307,
ferric iron/dipyridyl reacts more sensitively than the diphenylpicrylhydrazyl
reagent described by him previously[71]. The dipyridyl reagent is suitable for
determining compounds of low reactivity in concentrations down to 1-4ppm in
HB 307. The particular compounds studied by Koch[72] include, 4,4'thio-bis-
(-3methyl-6-tert-butylphenol),2,6,di-tert-butyl-4-methylphenol,tetrakis-
methylene-(3,5-di-test-butyl-4-hyroxy-hydrocinnamate)-methane,1,3,5-
trimethyl-2,4,6-tris-(3,5-di-tert-butyl-(4-hydroxy-benzyl)-benzene,1,1,3-tris-
(2-methyl-4-hydroxy-5-tert.butylphenyl)-butane and β-(3,5,di-tert-butyl-4-
hydroxy-phenyl)-propionic acid-octadecyl ester.

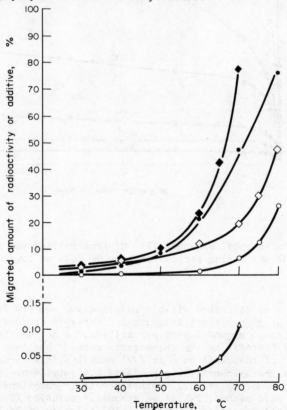

FIG.43 Migration of labelled additives (Ionox 330 o-o and stearamide ●-●) from
high density polyethylene film, Ionox 330 ◇ and n-butyl stearate ◆)
from polystyrene film and Avastab 17 MOK (△) from PVC film into fat
simulant HB 307 during a 10 day period at

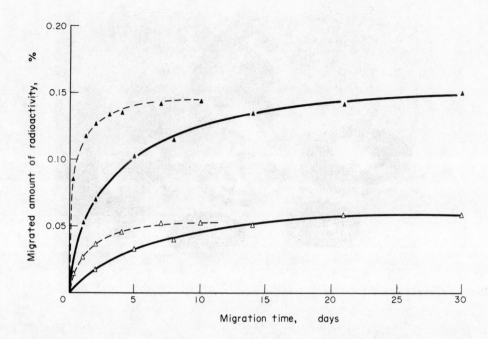

FIG.44   Effect of contact time on the migration of radioactivity from PVC test films
(Solvic, , Vinoflex,) containing ^{14}C-labelled tin stabilizer and
maintained in one-sided contact with fat simulant HB 307 at 20°C (△ -- ;
△ ——) and 40°C (▲ -- ; ▲ ——). The amount of radioactivity is
expressed as a percentage of the radioactivity of the original test film.

In this method, a solution (1 ml) containing 3 to 90µg of antioxidant per ml in
ethanol - 1,2-dichloroethane (7:3) is added to 10 ml of 30% HB 307 solution in
ethanol - 1,2-dichloroethane (7:3) in a test-tube. Then 0.5ml of 0.5%
ethanolic 2,2'-bipyridyl and 1ml of 0.2% ethanolic ferric chloride hexahydrate
added and the tube heated, in the dark, for 60 minutes in a water bath at 60°C,
then cooled in water at 20°C. the extinction of the solution is measured at
520nm in a 5-cm cell. Beer's law is obeyed for up to 10 to 30ppm of antioxidant, according to the compound. Some sulphur containing antioxidants can
be determined by this method, but with poorer sensitivity than by the
diphenylpicrylhydrazyl method.

Uhde et al[73] [74] have studied the migration of 4,4'thiobis-6-tert-butyl-m-
cresol (Santonox R) from plastics utensils into sunflower seed oil. Sunflower
seed oil that had been stored in vessels of polyethylene containing this
antioxidant was diluted (3:5) with pentane and extracted with acetonitrile
containing 5% of water. The concentrated acetonitrile extract (or an ethanol
solution of the residue on evaporation) was subjected to thin-layer
chromatography on Kieselgel with hexane-ethyl acetate (10:3) as solvent. To
detect the antioxidant (down to 0.1ppm) the plate was sprayed with 3,5-dichloro-
p-benzoquinonechlorimine solution. To determine the antioxidant, the zone at $R_F \simeq$
0.44 (located by means of iodine vapour) was removed and treated with fuming

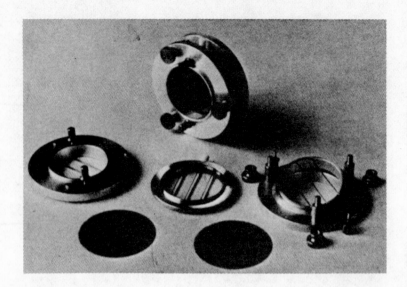

FIG.45 Migration Cell

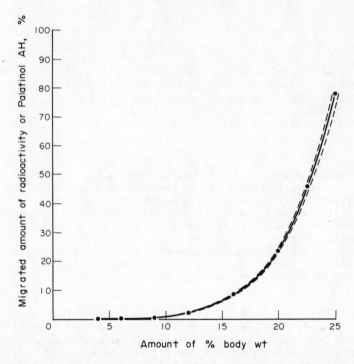

FIG.46 Mean migration of plasticizer di-(-2-ethyl-n-hexyl)phthalate from PVC test
films as a function of the plasticizer content. Broken lines indicate the
coefficient of variation of the single results about the mean.

nitric acid - sulphuric acid (1:1). The nitro-derivative of the antioxidant was determined in the product by polarography after the addition of urea and sodium acetate[74]. Alternatively, an aliquot of the original concentracted acetonitrile extract was treated with ethanol and diazotised sulphanilic acid, and the extinction of the resulting dye, measured at 480nm, was compared with that for a solution containing 10μg of antioxidant in acetonitrile, treated similarly.

Uhde and Waggon[75] also studied the migration of 2,6-di-tert-butyl-p-cresol from polystyrene, impact resistant polystyrene and polypropylene utensils. Samples of the utensils (10cm × 10cm × 1mm) containing less than 0.5% of antioxidant were immersed for 10 days at 45° in water, 3% acetic acid, 15% or 50% aqueous ethanol, heptane, and sunflower seed oil. The migration of the antioxidants from the plastics into the liquids was followed by the use of spectrophotometric or polarographic methods. The tests showed that there was little tendency for migration of the various antioxidants from the polystyrenes into the aqueous alcoholic or fatty liquids but there was considerable migration of 2,6-di-t-butyl-p-cresol from polypropylene into sunflower seed oil, and migration values were high whenever heptane was used.

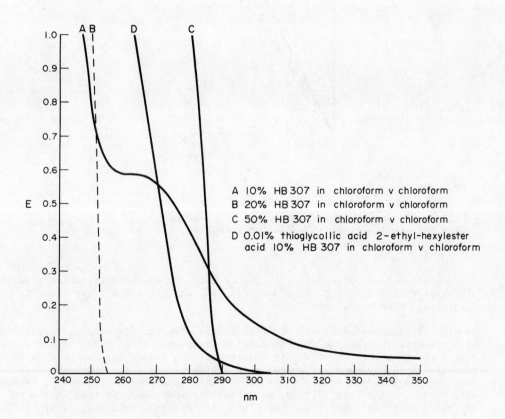

FIG.47 Ultraviolet absorption curves of thioglycollic acid-2-ethyl hexyl ester and HB 307 in chloroform.

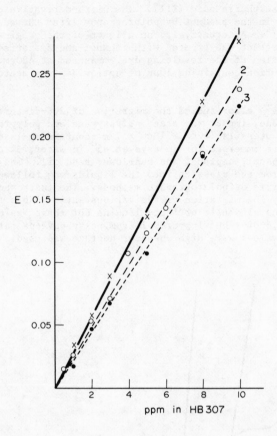

FIG.48   Calibration curves.   Ultraviolet spectroscopic determination in HB 307 of:

     (1) 2-(2'hydroxy-5'-methylphenyl)benzotriazole,
     (2) Thioethyleneglycol-bis-(βaminocrotonate,
     (3) 2-phenylindole.

The migration from polyethylene or PVC of hydroxyphenylbenzotriazoles used as ultraviolet absorbers into sunflower seed oil and linseed oil has been determined (Uhde and Waggon[117 118])

Samples of sunflower seed oil and linseed oil that had been stored in vessels of polyethylene or poly(vinyl chloride) containing 0.15 to 0.25% of the ultraviolet absorber were dissolved in cyclohexane and passed through columns of Kieselgel. Each column was washed with cyclohexane and the combined concentrated percolates were subjected to thin-layer chromatography on Kieselgel with heptane-chloroform (4:1) as solvent. The spots were located in 365-nm radiation or by spraying the dried plate with Prussian blue reagent or 2% Fast red salt AL solution. Semi-quantitative determinations were possible by comparing the size and intensity of the spots with those of standards. More exact determination was effected by polarography between -1.3 and -1.8 V vs. the mercury pool, the electrolyte consisting of 16ml of benzene, 12ml of perchloric acid and 4ml of water diluted to 100ml with ethanol. The $E_{\frac{1}{2}}$ value for 5-chloro-2-(5-t-butyl-6-hydroxy-m-tolyl)benzotriazole is -1.5V.

Alternatively, the oil sample was dissolved in isopropyl ether and the extinction was measured at 340, 343 or 353nm against a similar solution of the original untreated oil and referred to a calibration graph prepared with 1 to 50µg of the ultratiolet absorber added to 1g of oil[77].

Sampaolo et al[78] determined the specific migration of 2,2' methylene bis-(-6-tert-butyl-4-methylphenol) from rubber goods into ailimentary fats. They determined the antioxidant by the methods of Hilton[79] and Wadelin[80]. After extraction from styrene-butadiene, natural, butyl and nitrile rubbers into triolein or coconut oil by immersing discs of the rubber into the fat for 10 days at 40°C. Results of the two methods agreed well. The concentration of antioxidant in the extracts ranged from approximately 18 to 63 ppm, the largest amounts being extracted from natural rubber and the smallest amounts from nitrile rubber. Similar results were obtained for the migration of the antioxidant into heptane.

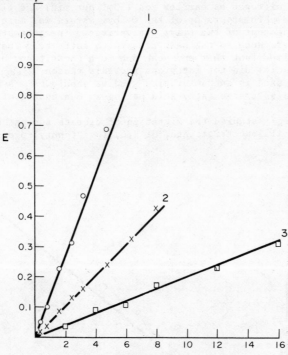

FIG.49   Photometric determination in HB 307 of (diphenyl picrylhydrazyl reagent):

(1)   2,2'methylene bis (-4-methyl-6-cyclohexyl phenol-1),

(2)   Thioglycollic acid-2ethylhexyl ester,

(3)   4,4'butylidene-bis-(3methyl-6-tert-butylphenol-1).

Piacentini[81] developed an indirect gas chromatographic method for the
determination of the migration of additives from rubber articles into olive
oil and coconut oil. Test pieces (25mm × 100mm × 0.5mm) of nitrile rubber
were weighed and suspended in olive or coconut oil; control pieces were
similarly suspended in air. After the desired time, the pieces were removed,
cleaned, dried and weighed. The total weight of material absorbed by the oil
from the rubber was derived by deducting the final weight from the sum of the
initial weight plus the weight of oil absorbed. To determine the weight of
oil absorbed, the pieces of rubber were heated under reflux with N-ethanolic
potassium hydroxide for 8 hours, and after acidification with hydrochloric acid
the liberated fatty acids were extracted with ethyl ether. The methyl esters
or the silyl derivatives were prepared and subjected to gas chromatography on,
respectively, a stainless-steel column (250cm × 4mm) packed with 15% of LAC
72S on Diatoport S (60 to 80 mesh) or on a similar column (180cm × 2mm) packed
with 10% of W 9S on Diatoport S (80 to 100 mesh). The columns were operated
at 200°C, with nitrogen as carrier gas (50ml per min) and flame ionisation
detection. The chromatography of the methyl esters was more accurate, but
less rapid, than that of the silyl derivatives. The chromatograms were
evaluated by reference to the peak area for a fatty acid characteristic of the
oil, it being important that any peak due to a constituent of the rubber
(e.g. stearic acid) did not interfere; for this reason, Piacentini[81] proposed
that the 'fat' used in such migration studies should be a synthetic triglyceride
prepared from a saturated fatty acid having an odd number of C atoms.

Bergner and Berg[82] studied the migration of citrate and phthalate plasticizers
from PVC and cellulose triacetate, of 2,6,di-tert-butyl-p-cresol from impact

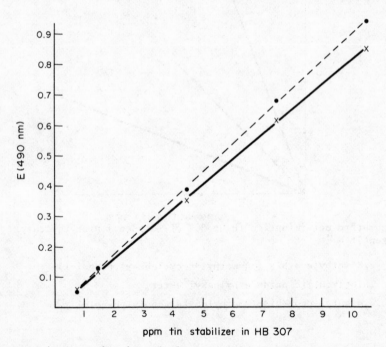

Fig.50   Photometric determination of di-n-octyltin stabilizers in HB 307:

    (a) Di-n-octyltin-bis-(2ethylhexyl-thioglycollate,
    (b) Di-n-octyltin maleate.

resistant polystyrene, of butylated hydroxy anisole from polyethylene, and of dioctyltin stabilizers from PVC into various organic solvents and into natural and synthetic triglycerides under various conditions of temperature and time.

Gas chromatography has been employed for the direct detection of the migration of phthalate plasticizers from plastics materials into fat and fatty foods, (Rohleder and Bruchhausen[83]). In this method a 7% solution of the sample, e.g. a solution of butter fat containing a plasticiser such as dibutyl phthalate) in acetone is cooled in a centrifuge-tube in a bath of ice-salt (3:1) to freeze out the greater part of the fat. The tube is centrifuged for 1 minute and the supernatant solution is decanted. This solution (2 or 5µl) is injected on to a pre-column (17 cm × 3mm) that is packed with Chromosorb G DMCS (80 to 100 mesh) coated with a mixture of SE-30 and dicyclohexyl phthalate and has been conditioned for 15 hours at 370°C in the presence of nitrogen. This pre-column adsorbs the remaining fat from the test solution and the plasticizer passes to the analytical gas chromatographic column (2metres × 3mm) packed with 4% of Silicone oil DC on Chromosorb G AW-DMCS (80 to 100mesh) and temperature programmed from 140° to 250°C at 22.5^{o} per minute with nitrogen as carrier gas (28ml per minute) and a flame ionisation detector. Down to 30ppm of plasticizers of high boiling point can be determined in fat with an error within ±6%. Rohleder and Bruchhausen[83] applied this method to cheese with a plastic outer coating.

6.4. Determination of organotin stabilizers in fats

Koch[84] has described a direct quantitative determination of di-n-octyltin compounds in fat simulant HB 307 using dithizone reagent. This method has a lower detection limit of 0.75ppm of the organotin compound. If the migration tests are carried out at a ratio of plastics surface (cm^2) to amount of fat simulant (g) of 5:1, then the detection limit for organotin stabilizers is 15µg/dm^2 (Fig.50). The same paper describes direct colorimetric methods for determining sodium alkyl sulphate, and sodium alkyl sulphonates in the 0.2-0.5 ppm concentration range (Fig.51) in HB 307 after reaction with methylene blue. Excellent calibration curves are obtained in these methods.

The extractability of labelled organotin compounds (di-n-octyl$\left[^{14}C\right]$tin-dithioglycollic acid-z-ethyl-n-hexyl ester) also other labelled compounds (1,3,5,trimethyl,2,4,6-tris(3,5-di-tert-butyl-4-hydroxy benzyl-$\left[^{14}C\right]$-benzol-Ionox 330, stearamide$\left[^{14}C\right]$, and n-butyl stearate$\left[^{14}C\right]$) from rigid PVC, low and high density polyethylene and polystyrene into mono, di and tri-glycerides has also been determined radiometrically (Figge[85]).

Figge and Zeman[86] have also studied the extractability of organotin compounds from rigid PVC using radiometric procedures. The organotin compounds studied included, di-n-octyltin-di-thioglycollic acid-2-ethyl hexyl ester, di-n-octyltin oxide, di-n-butyl tin dichloride, n-octylstannone, n-butylthiostannone, tri-n-octyltin fluoride, di-n-butyl-tin dilaurate, di-n-butyl tin dipropionate and di-n-octyltin maleate.

Figge and Koch[87] have studied the migration of Avastab TIMI8IFS (methyltin thioglycollic acid-2-ethyl-n-hexyl ester) from PVC into HB 307 fat simulant. Two preparations of this stabilizer with, respectively , the methyltin and the thioglycollic acid-2-ethyl-n-hexyl-ester ^{14}C labelled were incorporated into powdered polyvinyl chloride in amounts of 0.5, 1.0 and 1.5% by weight each. From the resulting rigid PVC mixtures compression-moulded films were made having specific radioactivities between 1.7 and 8.8 µCi/g. The even distribution of the radioactive quantities of stabilizer in the different

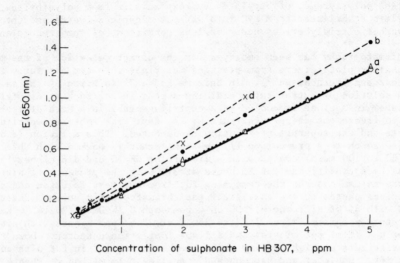

FIG.51 Photometric determination of anionic detergents in HB 307:

    (a) Statexan K1,
    (b) Sodium tridecane-1-sulphonate,
    (c) Sodium hexadecane-1-sulphonate,
    (d) Sodium dodecane-1-sulphate.

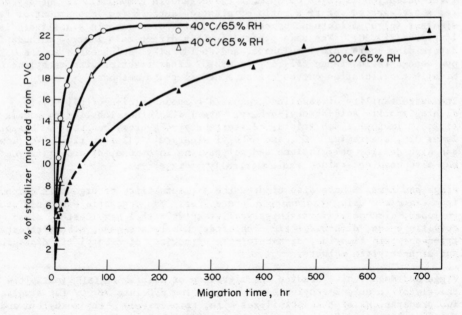

FIG.52 Extraction curve, migration of labelled Avastab TM181 from PVC into HB
    307 (1.5% additive in PVC film).

samples was checked by direct continuous radioanalytical measuring methods as well as by autoradiography and liquid scintillation counter.

In model tests the migration of methyl tin stabilizer and of its methyl-tin and thioglycollic acid-ester residues from rigid PVC into edible fats was checked radiometrically during 30 days at 20°C/65% relative humidity and 10 days at 40°C/65% relative humidity in one-sided contact as well as for 30 minutes at 70°C in all-round contact between the film samples and the fat simulant HB 307. It was found that under the same test conditions, despite an increasing stabilizer content of the film samples, the % migration of stabilizer as related to the total content of the films remains constant. However, the migration and extraction values depend on the different test conditions (Fig.52).

Assuming that the intact methyl tin stabilizer migrates from the rigid PVC into the fat simulant and that 10 dm^2 of PVC are in contact with 1kg of each simulating agent, for films with a stabilizer content of 1.5% by weight, migrate concentrations found in the simulant were: 0.18 and 0.35ppm after 30 days at 20°C, 0.14 and 0.15ppm after 10 days at 40°C and 0.044 and 0.11ppm after 30 minutes at 70°C. The migration/time curves show that with a prolonged testing time these concentrations do not increase.(Fig.53) Figge and Koch[87] also discuss the migration of hydrolysis products of the stabilizer.

In further work on the migration of Avastab TM181FS stabilizer from PVC, Figge and Bieber[88] study the migration rate from PVC into HB 307 of four methyl tin stabilizers of identical chemical composition, containing either monomethyl [^{14}C]-tin-tri-,di-methyl [^{14}C]-tin-di-, trimethyl [^{14}C]-tin-mono-thioglycolic acid-2-ethyl hexyl ester, or all three ^{14}C-labelled methyl tin compounds as radioactive indicators. These were incorporated into four identical powdered PVC mixtures in an amount of 1.5% by weight each. The resulting rigid PVC

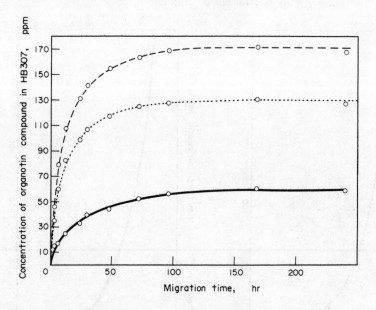

FIG.53 Extraction curve, migration of Avastab TM181MS(----o----), thioglycollic acid-2-ethylhexyl ester (...o...), methyl tin chloride (— o —) from PVC film into HB 307. Extraction temperature, 40°C; relative humidity, 65%; area of PVC film, 10dm^2;

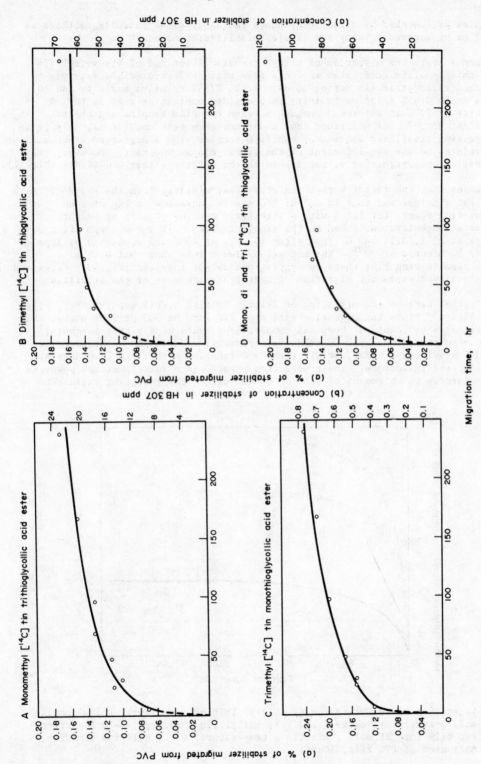

FIG. 54   Extraction curves at 40°C, 65% relative humidity. Mixtures of labelled methyltin stabilisers (methyltin-monothioglycollic acid-2-ethylhexyl ester) in PVC contacted with HB 307:
(a) % of labelled stabilisers migrated from PVC in contact with HB 307,
(b) concentration (PPB) of labelled stabilisers in HB 307 (10dm² PVC contacted with 1kg HB 307.

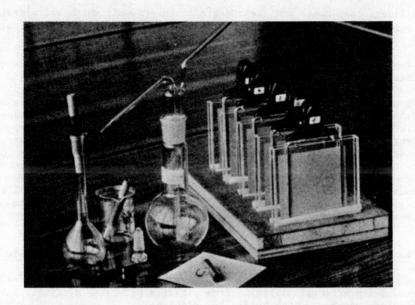

FIG.55   Migration chambers and other apparatus for the determination of total
         migrate.

mixtures were processed into compression-moulded films, the specific radio-
acitivities of which varied between 0.6 and 4.5μ Ci/g.

In model tests the migration of radioactive stabilizer components from the rigid
PVC films into the fat simulant HB 307 was determined radiometrically over a
period of 10 days during which the films were stored at 40°C/65% relative
humidity, one side of the film being in contact with the simulant. Assuming
that the intact stabilizer components migrate, the results show that fat-
containing food products packed and stored in rigid PVC materials stabilized
with Avastab TM 181 FS will contain not more than 1ppb trimethyl-tin-mono-,
73ppb dimethyl-tin-di- and 39ppb monomethyl-tin-tri-thioglycolate. Assuming
that the methyl tin thioglycolates are converted into the methyl tin chlorides
before or during migration, the corresponding concentrations are 0.5ppb
trimethyl-tin-mono-, 29ppb dimethyl-tin-di- and 13ppb monomethyl-tin-trichloride.
The migration/time curves show that these concentrations hardly increase on
prolonging the test period. Figge and Bieber[88] also found that irrespective of
the duration of any heat treatment given to the PVC the amounts of trimethyl
tin compounds present in stabilized rigid PVC materials never exceed those
originally added with the methyl tin stabilizers.

Figge[89] examined the migration of three labelled methyltin stabilizers from
PVC into HB 307. The three methyl tin stabilizers of identical chemical
composition were incorporated into rigid PVC film in amounts of 0.5, 1.0
and 1.5 wl.%. These stabilizers contained as radioactive indicators either
monomethyl[^{14}C]-tin-tri-, dimethyl [^{14}C]-tin-di-, trimethyl[^{14}C]-tin-monothio-
glycolic acid-2-ethyl hexyl ester or all three stabilizer components which
were ^{14}C-labelled in the methyl tin or thioglycolate residues. In model tests
these film samples were in one-side contact with HB 307 for 30 days at 20°C/65%
relative humidity and for 10 days at 40°C relative humidity or immersed in the
fat simulant for 30 minutes at 70°C. The amounts of methyl tin stabilizers,

stabilizers components and their degradation products which had migrated from the rigid PVC into the simulant during these contact times were calculated from radio-analytical data.

The results show that (on the assumption that the stabilizer components migrate as intact molecules) fat-containing foods packed and stored in rigid PVC will not contain more than 1ppb trimethyl-tin-mono-, 73ppb dimethyl-tin-di- and 39ppb monomethyl-tin-trithioglycolic acid ester. Assuming that the methyl-tin-thioglycolates are transformed into the methyl chlorides and thioglycolates before or during their migration into fat-containing foods, the respective concentrations are 0.5ppb trimethyl-tin-mono-, 29ppb dimethyl-tin-di- and 13ppb monomethyl-tin-trichloride. The migration/time curves show that prolongation of test period gives practically no further increase in these concentrations, (Fig.54).

Methods have been described for the determination of the extractability of dioctyl-s,s'bis-(iso-octylmercapto)acetate stabilizers from PVC into sunflower seed oil (Adcock and Hope[17]).

6.5. The Concept of Total Migration of Additives from Plastics into Edible Fats

Figge[90] [91] [92] and Figge and Koch [93] have carried out extensive studies of the determination of total migration from plastics packaging materials into edible fats using a ^{14}C-labelled fat simulant.

Migration is the term used for the transfer of additives, monomers and other compounds under conditions of filling or storage (e.g. at $20^{\circ}C$ and 65% relative humidity) from packaging materials into the products they contain or into simulants of such products. Transfer of a particular compounds of toxicological interest is designated 'specific migration' whereas total migration refers to the transfer of all mobile packaging components.

Unlike tests for specific migration, determination of the total migrate does not involve any direct toxicological considerations because both toxic substances and physiologically harmless packaging components are included. This test is therefore used at present only for checking new batches of already approved packaging materials, for which the total migration limits are known to the manufacturers. However, determining the total migrate from new packaging materials awaiting approval could give an important indication of total contamination and thus of the possible adulteration of the packed foodstuffs. Nevertheless, it has generally been considered that the determination of total migration is inadequate for a final physiological assessment of a new packaging material.

The Dutch Health Authorities have presented interesting proposals for the standardization and simplification of the analytical procedures for packaging-materials approvals (Aldershoff[94]), according to which the total migrate could serve as a basis for physiological assessment. It is suggested that approval of an additive for any type of packaging should be given only if the amount of additive migrating from the final pack into the food contained in it does not exceed a maximum determined as acceptable on the basis of animal trials. This means that the present limit on the amount of an additive in the packaging material would be replaced by a maximum allowable quantity of additive migrating into the foodstuff. A limit of 60ppm (60mg/kg food) has been proposed for the tolerable total migrate in packaged foods.

Assuming a contact area of $5dm^2$/kg between the packaging material and the packaged food, the admissable total migrate is thus to be limited to $12mg/dm^2$

of the packaging surface. Exceptions to this rule are considered necessary
in the case of plasticized PVC, paper, cellophane and rubber.

The German Federal Ministry of Health (Bundesgesundheitsamt) considers,
however, that in view of the trend towards small packs, the total amount of
migratable material should be fixed at a lower level of 6mg/dm^2 packaging-
material surface and this implies an accuracy in analytical methods of 0.5mg
total migrate/dm^2 of food packing surface.

Figge[90] considered various methods whereby this analysis could be achieved
for fatty extractants.

Methods in which volatile solvents like n-heptane and diethyl ether are used
as fat simulants and the total migrate is determined in the evaporation
residue (Baumgartner[95]; Federal Health Office, Berne[96]; Italian Ministry of
Health[97]; US Code of Federal Regulations[98] [99]) are not appropriate for
reasons outlined by Figge and Piater[100]. The remaining methods are indirect,
depending on the determination of the loss of migratable components from a
packaging material in contact with a test fat. Of two approaches described
in the literature, one is too inaccurate to be of value (BITMP (Bureaux
Internationaux Techniques des Matieres Plastiques[101]); Brugger[102]: de Wilde[103]
Fluckiger and Rentsch[104]; Robinson-Gornhardt[105] [106]; Laboratoire cantonal de
Berne[107]). The second, more promising, approach involves weighing a packaging-
material sample before and after storage in a test fat under defined test
conditions. The difference between the two weights gives the total weight of
the migrate, provided the test fat remaining in and on the packaging-material
sample after storage is taken into account (BITMP[101]). Methods based on this
principle have the advantage that the same packaging-material sample is used
in all steps of the investigation. However, the analytical methods currently
used to determine the absorption of fat by the test film are relatively
complicated and inaccurate (BITMP[108]; Pfab[109]; van Battum and Rijk[110];
Wildbrett, Evers and Kiermeier[111]; Koch[112]). As a consequence of this Figge[90]
developed a generally applicable ratio-tracer method, by which the total
amount of material that has migrated into the fat simulant HB 307 (Chapter 2),
(Figge[113]; Figge, Eder and Piater[114]), can be estimated indirectly from the
decrease in weight of the packaging material being tested. A representative
sample of the packaging material is weighed before and after storage in the
radioactively-labelled fat simulant (HB 307- ^{14}C *) and the amount of HB 307
^{14}C retained in and on the sample in spite of careful cleaning is determined
by radio-analysis. The suitability of the synthetic standard triglyceride
mixture, HB 307, as a fat simulant is indicated by Table 19 which shows that
the amounts of additives migrating from various test films into HB 307 are
never more than 1.8 times as great as the values for the reference fats, Biskin,
coconut oil and butter. Moreover, additive migration from plastics into
Biskin corresponds with that into margarine, olive and sunflower oils and
other edible oils (Figge[115]; Figge and Piater[116]; Piater and Figge[117];
vom Bruck, Figge, Piater and Wolf[118]).

This approach is a distinct improvement on that involving direct extraction of
the plastic with solvents such as methanol, diethyl ether or heptane followed
by removal of solvents from the extract at 40°C and 12 Torr and weighing.
Piater and Figge[117] showed that when the dry residues of the extraction
solutions from films of rigid PVC, polystyrene, high density and low density
polyethylene, extracted with methanol, diethyl ether and n-heptane (5 hours
65 or 35°C) are compared with the quantities of ^{14}C-labelled additives
contained in these extracts and those which within 60 days have migrated into
sunflower seed oil, the total extract is in general not conclusive of the
amount of additives extracted by solvents or migrated into edible oil. For

low density-PE and methanol for instance it is 2.5 times higher and in the
case of PVC and diethyl ether it is as much as 2280 times higher than the
total amount of all radioactive additives, which with 60 days at $20^{\circ}C$ have
migrated into sunflower seed oil. In this case PVC contained, however,
additionally 1.0% of non-radioactively labelled lubricants which contributed
to the total extract.

The principles of the method for determining total migration into HB 307-^{14}C
described by Figge[90] are discussed below.

The total migrate (GM) is calculated from the radio-analytically determined
amount (mg) of fat absorbed (F_p) and the weight (mg) of the packaging-material
sample before storage (Gv) and after storage (Gn) in HB 307-^{14}C (equation I):

$$GM = Gv - (Gn - Fp) \, (mg) \tag{I}$$

The advantages offered by this procedure are only realized if the determination
of the fat absorption (Fp) by the test material is carried out rapidly and
without interference and additional corrections.

HB 307 labelled with ^{14}C for use as a tracer substance in this context can
reasonably be characterized only by its specific radioactivity, S_F, expressed
in nCi or pCi/mg. Characterization by nCi/mmole is less accurate and is only
possible if the mean molar mass of all the triglycerides in the fat simulant
is known.

On the other hand, it must be recognized that triglycerides of different
molecular size penetrate into plastics to differing degrees (Figge[115]). It
is therefore to be expected that from a triglyceride mixture like HB 307 the
low-molecular triglycerides will migrate preferentially into the test materials,
so that if the triglycerides of the fat simulant were labelled exclusively
in their glycerol residues or only in the acyl residues, the specific radioactivity, S_F, of the original HB 307- ^{14}C , which is considered to serve as
the operand, would not be identical with the specific radioactivity, S_{Fp}, of
the simulant fraction, F_p, migrating into the test material. Consequently,
during the determination of the fat absorption, F_p, an intentional systematic
error would be introduced, differing from one packaging material to another.
An accurate and rapid determination of the fat absorption, F_p, without the
necessity of correction is possible by this radio-tracer method only when
both the glycerol residue used for synthesizing the HB 307- ^{14}C and each
acyl residue possess radioactivity proportional to their respective molar
masses.

It is a prerequisite that the radioactivity, A_{Fp}(nCi), migrating into the
test material with the simulant fraction, F_p, is directly proportional to
F_p:

$$A_{Fp} = S_{Fp} \cdot F_p \, (nCi) \tag{II}$$

On the other hand:

$$A_{Fp} = f_1 s_1 + f_2 s_2 + f_3 s_3 + \ldots f_n S_n \, (nCi) \tag{III}$$

if f_i is the mass and S_i the specific radioactivity (nCi/mg) of the triglycerides
with the same molecular weight present in the simulant faction, F_p.

Equations II and III are then satisfied if

$$S_{Fp} \cdot F_p = f_1 S_1 + f_2 S_2 + f_3 S_3 + \ldots f_n S_n \, (nCi) \tag{IV}$$

TABLE 19

Comparison of the amounts of additive migrating from different test films into edible fats and the fat simulant HB 307 during one-sided contact for 60 days at 20°C

Test film*	Identity and concn (%,w/w) of labelled additive	Proportion of radioactivity or additive migrating into				Ratio R† for		
		Biskin	Coconut Oil	Butter	HB 307	Biskin	Coconut Oil	Butter
Rigid PVC	Irgastab 17 MOK-[^{14}C]‡(1.5)	0.009	0.014	0.017	0.016	1.8	1.1	1.0
HD polyethylene	Ionox 330-[^{14}C]§(1.0)	0.090	0.098	0.120	0.0	1.6	1.4	1.2
	Stearic acid[1-^{14}C] amide (0.2)	0.80	0.96	1.05	1.36	1.7	1.4	1.3
Polystyrene	Ionox 330-[^{14}C](2.0)	2.08	2.53	3.07	3.05	1.5	1.2	1.0
	n-Butyl stearate[1-^{14}C](0.5)	5.20	5.61	7.11	7.57	1.5	1.4	1.1

* Figge et al[114]

† R = $\dfrac{\text{amount of additive migrating into fat simulant HB 307}}{\text{amount of additive migrating into Biskin, coconut oil or butter}}$

‡ Di-n-octyl[1-^{14}C]-tin-bis-(2-ethylhexylthioglycollate) (Figge[52])

§ 1,3,5-Trimethyl-2,4-tris-(3,5-di-tert-butyl-4-hydroxybenzyl[^{14}C]) benzene (Figge[53])

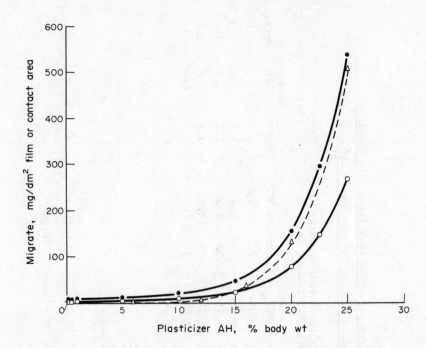

FIG.56   Influence of plasticizer content of PVCtest films on the specific migration
         (SM;) of di-(2-ethyl-n-hexyl)phthalate calculated on contact area   △
         total migration (GM) calculated on the size of film (●), and on the
         contact area (0), into the fat simulant HB 307- ^{14}C

known specific radioactivity, S_F, of the original fat simulant HB 307-^{14}C
in which case

$$\frac{A_{Fp}}{S_F} = \frac{A_{Fp}}{S_{Fp}} = F_p \text{(mg)} \tag{V}$$

As mentioned before, this aim is only reached if the glycerol residue and
all the acyl residues contributing to the synthesis of HB 307- ^{14}C possess
the same specific radioactivity, s(nCi/mg), so that each triglyceride
molecule in the simulant has a level of radioactivity, A_{Tr}, proportional
to its molar mass:

$$A_{Tr} = s(m_{GI} + m_{Ac(1)} + m_{Ac(2)} + m_{Ac(23)} \tag{VI}$$

and $s = S_{Fp} = S_F$; m_{G1} being the mass of the glycerol residue and $m_{Ac(1-3)}$
the individual masses of the three acyl residues in the triglyceride molecule.

Migration-test procedure with plastics films.   A specimen 1 dm^2 in size is
punched out from the packaging film using a square-puncher.   Surface
contamination is cleaned from the test film by careful rubbing with foamed

plastics previously extracted three times with fresh supernatant ethanol at 60°C for 30 minutes. It is then kept for 24 hours at 20°C and 65% relative humidity and weighed accurately (Gv). For a further characterization of the test film, the mean thickness, D, can be determined. During this preparative work, the migration cell is packed with 120g fat simulant, HB 307- ^{14}C , which is equilibrated at 40°C. The cell consists of a glass vessel 1.3cm high, 12cm long and 1cm wide. As illustrated in Fig. 55 the test film is fixed in a clamp and stored for 10 days in a bath of fat maintained at 40°C.

After storage, the test film is freed as far as possible from adhering test fat by careful dabbing with extracted foamed plastics at 40°C and is placed on foamed plastics. The specimen is than placed in the weighing sleeve, equilibrated for 24 hours at 20°C and 65% relative humidity and is weighed (Gn). First, the total weight of sleeve and film is determined, and then the sample is pushed into a 100-ml measuring flask with forceps and the empty sleeve is weighed alone.

The test film is then dissolved in the measuring flask, and the flask is filled up to the mark. Aliquots of this solution, generally five samples each of 2.0ml, are measured in a suitable scintillation liquid using a liquid scintillation spectrometer. Since scintillation counting is a statistical measuring procedure, the measuring accuracy and detection limit depend mainly on the measuring time, i.e. long measuring times guarantee a high degree of accuracy. The radioactivity, A_{Fp}, of the fat-containing test film, in nCi or pCi, can be calculated directly from the mean of the individual measurements.

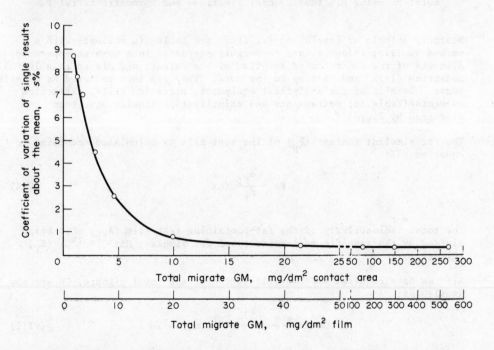

FIG.57 Coefficient of variation of the single results about the mean (5%) for the radio-traced method as a function of the total migration (Gm) determined with the fat simulant HB-307- ^{14}C

$$(5\% = \frac{\text{standard deviation}}{\text{mean value for 5 determinations}} \cdot 100$$

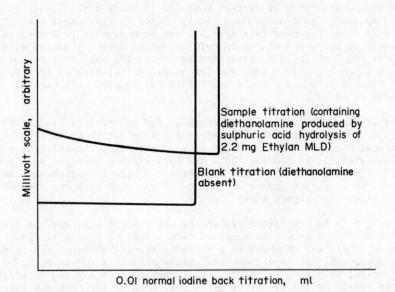

FIG. 58 Potentiometric titration of sodium arsenite with standard iodine
         solution using platinum/calomel electrode and automatic titrator.

Scarcely soluble or insoluble test films are boiled in solvents with a
marked swelling effect or are thoroughly extracted in a Soxhlet apparatus.
Aliquots of the concentrated solution of the extract are placed in a 100-ml
measuring flask and made up to the mark. They are then measured as described
above. Details of the analytical equipment, migration cells, extraction
solvents (Table 19) extractants and scintillation liquids have been
discussed by Figge[119].

The fat simulant content (F_p) of the test film is calculated according to
equation VII:

$$Fp = \frac{A_{Fp}}{S_F} \ (mg) \tag{VII}$$

the total radioactivity of the fat-containing test film $(A_{Fp}$, nCi$)$ being
divided by the specific radioactivity of fat simulant HB 307- ^{14}C $(S_F$,
nCi/mg$)$.

All the data required for the calculation of the total migrate, GM are now
available:

$$GM = \frac{Gv - (Gn - Fp)}{KF} \ (mg/dm^2) \tag{VIII}$$

where Gv is the weight (mg) of test film before and Gn the weight (mg) of
test film after storage in HB 307- ^{14}C , KF is the contact area (dm^2)
between test film and fat and Fp is the content (mg) of test fat in the
stored test film. Equation VIII is free of correction terms since the radio-

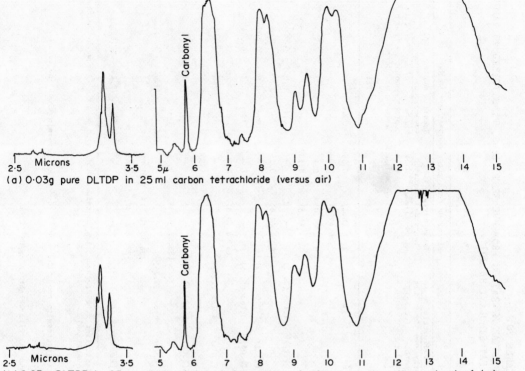

(a) 0·03g pure DLTDP in 25 ml carbon tetrachloride (versus air)

(b) 0·03g DLTDP in 25 ml carbon tetrachloride versus air found in the ether extract of (a)
distilled water B.P.F. extractant (b) 1·1 ethanol: water B.P.F. extractant (c) 5% sodium carbonate
B.T.F. extractant (d) 5% citric acid B.P.F. extractant (all after heating extractant for 10 days
at 60°C)

FIG. 59   Infrared spectra of ether extracts of solutions of dilauryl
          thiodipropionate in the British Plastics Federation extractants.

tracer method the determination of blank values is unnecessary.

Table 20 summarises a series of results on various PVC films tested by this
radio-tracer method using pressed PVC films containing 0-25% (w/w) of the
plasticizer (di-2ethyl-n-hexyl)phthalate.   Some of the test films contained,
^{14}C-labelled plasticizer so that both the total migration and the specific
transfer of the plasticizer into the fat simulant HB 307 could be determined
and related to the plasticizer content of the test film.   Conditions were
standardized, so the values obtained were directly comparable.

The total migration during all-sided contact and the specific migration of
plasticizer from one-sided contact of the test films with the fat simulant
HB 307 after a contact time of 10 days at 40°C appear in the right half of
Table 20.   From unplasticized PVC film, the total migrate amounted to 2.06
mg/dm^2 film of 1.03 mg/dm^2 contact area.   Increases of 5% in the plasticizer
content of the film to provide concentrations of 5, 10, 15, 20 and 25%
led to increases in the amounts of total migrate of 7.2, 10.7, 23.1, 112.6
and 382.6 mg/dm^2 film, respectively.   The increase in total migration thus
becomes larger the higher the plasticizer content of the film, as is also
the case with the specific migration of plasticizer from PVC films into

TABLE 20.

SPECIFIC MIGRATION OF DI-(2 ETHYL-N-HEXYL) PHTHALATE AND TOTAL MIGRATION FROM PVC TEST FILMS, PLASTICIZED TO VARYING DEGREES, INTO FAT SIMULANT HB 307

	Characteristics of PVC test films*					Migration data after contact for 10 days at 40°C				
Content of di-(2-ethyl-n-hexyl) phthalate (% w/w)	No. of determinations (n)...	Thickness of film (μm)‡	Weight of film (mg/dm²)‡	Specific radioactivity of di-(2-ethyl-n-hexyl) phthalate [^{14}C]† (μCi/g)‡	Test film (μCi/g)‡	Total migrate (GM) (two-sided contact) mg/dm² film‡	% of film weight§	Specific migrate (SM) (one-sided contact) mg/dm² contact area	% of amount of additive in film	% of film weight§
	50	50	5	10	40	5				
0.00		235 (5.1)	3442.97 (2.7)	–	–	2.06 (8.7)	0.060	–	–	–
0.25		244 (1.8)	3447.86 (4.9)	–	–	2.76 (7.8)	0.080	–	–	–
0.50		246 (1.2)	3349.48 (0.5)	–	–	3.72 (7.0)	0.111	–	–	–
1.0		243 (4.1)	3257.91 (3.7)	–	–	5.94 (4.5)	0.182	–	–	–
4.0		222 (7.3)	2990.3 (3.0)	104.21 (1.17)	4.139 (2.71)	–	–	0.011	0.009	0.0004
5.0		234 (5.3)	3111.46 (3.7)	–	–	9.24 (2.6)	0.297	–	–	–
6.0		224 (11.2)	2994.6 (3.0)	70.92 (1.11)	4.225 (1.24)	–	–	0.078	0.043	0.0026
9.0		218 (11.8)	3003.2 (2.8)	34.94 (1.06)	3.162 (1.96)	–	–	1.324	0.58	0.044
10.0		226 (2.9)	2933.58 (1.6)	–	–	19.94 (0.8)	0.679	–	–	–
12.0		220 (7.0)	2960.3 (3.0)	34.94 (1.06)	4.155 (1.57)	–	–	7.21	2.04	0.244
15.0		215 (8.8)	2824.03 (8.4)	–	–	43.00 (0.40)	1.53	–	–	–
16.0		210 (5.5)	2758.5 (2.7)	34.94 (1.06)	5.823 (2.07)	–	–	38.26	8.30	1.39
20.0		212 (2.6)	2725.20 (1.6)	–	–	155.62 (0.34)	5.71	–	–	–
		216 (5.6)	2819.5 (2.3)	34.94 (1.06)	6.878 (2.24)	–	–	132.72	23.91	4.71
22.5		221 (4.5)	2684.96 (1.6)	–	–	296.68 (0.31)	11.05	–	–	–
25.0		205 (7.0)	2631.20 (5.9)	–	–	538.26 (0.32)	20.46	–	–	–
		213 (4.8)	2849.1 (2.7)	34.94 (1.06)	8.617 (1.58)	–	–	510.52	72.48	17.92

*Vinoflex 503 (supplied by BASF, Ludwigshafen). In addition to the plasticizer, the pressed films contained 0.5% (w/w) Wachs E (Farbwerke Hoechst, Frankfurt/M.) and 0.5% (w/w) stabilizer C (Farbenfabriken Bayer AG, Leverkusen).

†Di-(2-ethyl-n-hexyl) [7,8-^{14}C]phthalate.

‡Values in parentheses are the coefficients of variation (s%) of the single results about the mean of the no. of determinations indicated (s% = $\frac{\text{standard deviation}}{\text{mean value}}$ × 100).

§Calculated from GM in mg/dm² film or from SM in mg/dm² contact area and the film weight in mg/dm² film.

HB 307. This clearly demonstrated in Fig.56 in which the specific migration
of the plasticizer and the total migration into HB 307 are plotted as a
function of the plasticizer content of the PVC test film.

In addition to the increasing steepness of the migration curves for PVC
films containing more than 15% plasticizer, this graph also shows the close
similarity between the values for total migration from two-sided contact and
for specific migration of the plasticizer fron one-sided contact of the test
film with the fat simulant over this range of plasticizer concentrations.
This indicates that in a 10 day period at $40^{o}C$, a PVC film containing more
than 15% plasticizer imparts approximately the same amount of plasticizer
to HB 307 whether the contact is one-sided or two-sided. Consequently, the
total migrate from a $1dm^2$ piece of a highly plasticized PVC film should not
be halved to obtain the value for a contact area of $1dm^2$. It can in fact
be seen from Fig.56 that the curve obtained by halving the total migration
values in this way and plotting them against the plasticizer content of the
films does not conform to the actual migration as indicated by the curve of
the specific migration of plasticizer. Halving of the total migration values
is only appropriate if the test films are not swollen by the test fat, or are
only swollen at the surface.

Five determinations of the total migrate were carried out for each test film,
and from the individual results the mean total migrate and subsequently
the coefficient of variation of the single results about the mean were calculated.
In Fig.57 this coefficient of variation of the single results has been plotted
as a function of the mean total migrate determined with fat simulant HB 307-
^{14}C . In the case of total migrates greater than $25mg/dm^2$ contact area or
$50mg/dm^2$ film, this coefficient of variation amounts consistently to about
0.3%. In the range of the internationally discussed thresholds for total
migrate of 6 and $12mg/dm^2$ packaging material surface, a coefficient of
variation of about 2 and 0.6%, respectively, must be taken into account.
With a total migrate of $1mg/dm^2$ contact area, this error amounts to some 9%,
but even this is a relatively small error if one consider the   difficulties
of weighing the test materials before and after storage in the test fat.

In addition to these experiments on PVC test films containing different
concentrations of plasticizer, Figge[90] determined the total migrates from
two different low-density polyethylenes, from impact-resistant polystyrene and
from polyvinylidene chloride into fat simulant HB 307- ^{14}C . Table 21
lists the characteristics of the test materials and the migration results.
In all cases the coefficient of variation of the single determinations about
the mean was of the order of magnitude to be expected from the amount of
total migrate.

As discussed above, Figge[90] pointed out that triglycerides of different
molecular size penetrate into plastics to different degrees (Figge[115]) and
that it is therefore to be expected that from a triglyceride mixture like
HB 307 the low-molecular weight triglycerides will migrate preferentially
into the test plastics in determinations of total migration with the
consequent risk of error in the determination of this factor is not allowed
for. More recently, Koch and Figge[62] have confirmed this finding by gas
chromatography. Sunflowerseed oil and synthetic triglyceride mixture HB 307
were allowed to come into contact with rubber, low-density and high-density
polyethylene, polystyrene and rigid and plasticized PVC. The fat which
had migrated into the plastics was subsequently extracted from them with an
organic solvent and the composition of the extracted fat and of the original
fat compared by gas chromatography. In all cases an increase in the
concentration was found in favour of the low molecular weight triglycerides.

TABLE 21

Total migration (GM) from different plastics films into fat simulant HB 307

Type of plastics*	Trade name	Characteristics of test films			Total migrate(GM) after 10 days at 40°C and two-sided contact	
		No. of determinations (n)...	Thickness of film (μm)	Weight of film (mg/dm²)	mg/dm² contact area	% of weight of film†
			50	5	5	
LD-polyethylene	Lupolen 1810 H‡		103(5.8)	1003.44(6.3)	4.83(3.21)	0.481
	Lupolen 1840 D‡		88(15.4)	849.55(14.7)	3.19(3.95)	0.375
Impact-resistant polystyrene	476 L‡		104(2.3)	1053.32(2.3)	1.33(10.53)	0.126
Polyvinylidene chloride§	—		104(6.2)	1640.98(3.6)	33.09(0.51)	2.02

*   The exact composition of the extruded films was not known.

†   Calculated from GM in mg/dm² contact area and the film weight in mg/dm² film.

‡   Supplied by BASF, Ludwigshafen.

§   Containing 3% (w/w) dibutyl sebacate and 10% (w/w) Palamoll 646, a polyester of adipic acid and butane-1,3- and -1,4-diols supplied by BASF, Ludwigshafen.

Values in parentheses are the coefficients of variation (s%) of the single results about the mean of the number of determinations indicated.

The concentrations of linoleic acid had increased in the fat which had migrated into the rubber. In the case of all the other plastics examined the concentration of oleic acid in the fat which had migrated into the plastic had increased over the concentration present in the original fat. Such factors will consequently lead to errors in all methods of total migrate determination which are based on an assessment of individual components of the fat which have migrated into the plastic specimen. Koch and Figge[62], in this work, confirmed the conclusion reached earlier (Figge[90], see above) that the only procedure which is not affected by this phenomenon is the radiotracer method using HB 307 [14]C .

Koch and Kröhn[120] have described two further methods for the determination of the total migration from plastics into fats–based on enzymatic glycerol determination and colormetric glycerol determination using chromotropic acid and on gas chromatography and have compared results obtained by these methods with those obtained by methods described by Pfab[121] and van Battium and Rijk[122] and by the Figge[90] referee method using ^{14}C labelled fat simulant (see above). Koch and Kröhn[120] compared the four methods on the basis of susceptibility to interference and speed of analysis. The enzymatic glycerol determination of the amount (F_p) of fat simulant migrated into polystyrene and polyethylene is almost as lengthy as the chromotropic acid method. However, the enzymatic method is less susceptible to interferences. The determination of F_p by direct gas chromatography of the triglycerides on 1.2m x 2mm column of 40% polyethylene glycol A on Chromosorb G-AW-DMCS is less susceptible to inferences than that by the gas chromatography of the fatty acid methyl esters. This method was also the least time consuming of the four methods investigated.

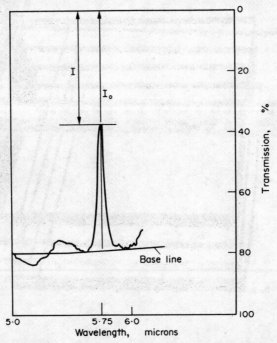

FIG.60 Infrared spectrum of a solution of dilaurylthiodipropionate in carbon tetrachloride showing the measurements required for determining the absorbance at the 5.75micron carbonyl peak.

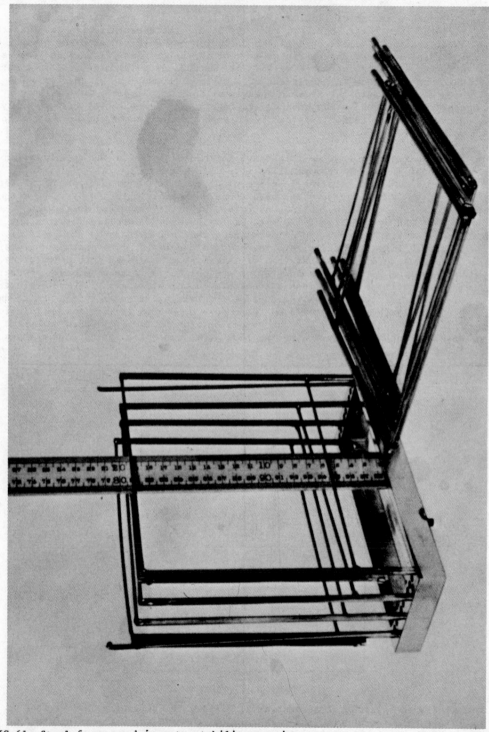

FIG.61   Steel frame used in extractability testing.

Chapter 7

Determination of Additives and their Degradation Products in Aqueous and in Simple Hydrocarbon Extractants

As discussed in Chapter 4.2, it is a fact that the analyst concerned with the analysis of additives in either synthetic extractants or foodstuffs may occasionally find that his problem is simple in that he has only to determine one substance without interferences and at an analysible concentration in a range of extractants. In practical circumstances, however, the problem is not generally as simple as this. Other additives or adventicious polymer impurities which have also extracted from the polymer into the extractant may be present and this frequently causes complications which the analyst has to circumvent. Also, of course, in many cases, analysis is required for more than one additive and this may necessitate the adoption of a separation technique prior to carrying out the final analysis. A particular circumstance where such problems manifest themselves is in the analysis of extractants of polymers in which complete or partial additive degradation has occured either during polymer processing or during its service life (eg. exposure to sunlight) or during the extraction test itself (e.g. hydrolysis of extracted additives by aqueous extractants). As such degradation products might themselves have toxicological properties it might be deemed to be necessary to carry out analysis for them as well as for the undegraded additive. Even if this is not considered necessary the analyst must be aware of any such degradation processes so that due allowance can be made for any interfering effects they may exert on the determination of the undegraded form of the additive or on the determination of any other substance which is to be analysed for in the extractant.

In addition to these considerations, there is also the rather more estoeric possibility of reaction between the extracted additive or its degradation products with a component of the extractant liquid to form compounds of different toxicology to the original additive. This factor should particularly be taken into account when dealing with edible oil types of extractants where distinct possibilities exist for reaction between migrated additives and components of the oil.

Instances of the possibility of a degradation of an additive and its effect on the design of the analytical procedure are supported below by means of two examples. The first of these is concerned with the antistatic additive lauric diethanolamide which has been used in foodgrade polyolefin and polystyrene formulations. This compound, upon migration from the plastic into aqueous extractant liquids hydrolyses quite readily to lauric acid and diethanolamine:

$$C_{11}H_{23}CON(CH_2CH_2OH)_2 + H_2O = C_{11}H_{23}COOH + HN(CH_2CH_2OH)_2$$

In fact any of this additive which extracts from a polymer into distilled water at $60^{\circ}C$ is hydrolysed fairly completely within a few days. The analytical problem, resolves itself, therefore, into the determination of traces of diethanolamine degradation product in the presence of relatively small concentrations of lauric diethanolamide. A method for the determination of lauric diethanolamide and diethanolamine in the aqueous and alcoholic extraction liquids of the British Plastics Federation and in liquid paraffin is described below.

These methods are considered in some detail as they illustrate well the amount of method development that is sometimes required to achieve the required analysis.

Lauric diethanolamide is a fairly unreactive substance. A likely approach to the problem of determining low concentrations of this substance involved hydrolysing it to a diethanolamine and fatty acid and determining the former by a conventional iodometric method. The lauric diethanolamide content of the extractant could then be calculated from the amount of diethanolamine produced upon complete hydrolysis. It is more appropriate to determine diethanolamine rather than the fatty acid, as it was possible that the extractant could contain fatty acids originating from sources other than hydrolysis of the dialkanolamide (e.g. free fatty acids or their metal salts or fatty acid esters, all of which might be present in the original polymer).

The required sensitivity of the analytical procedure is indicated by the following considerations. Under the extractability test conditions proposed by the British Plastics Federation on thin films (<0.020 inch) of polymer containing 0.03% w/w of additive, each cubic centimetre volume of plastic is contacted with $20cm^3$ of the extraction liquid. Thus, if all the additive present in the original polymer film migrates during the extraction test into the extraction liquid, at the end of the test this liquid will contain only approximately 15ppm of additive. Consequently it was necessary to devise a procedure for determining extracted polymer additive in each of the extractants in amounts down to 3 parts per million.

Lauric diethanolamide does not react with periodic acid in the presence of 0.03 normal sulphuric acid. To estimate lauric diethanolamide it is first necessary to hydrolyse it to diethanolamine, which can then be determined by the periodic acid method. Tests to determine the conditions necessary to completely hydrolyse lauric diethanolamide (Table 22) showed that it hydrolyses quite slowly. In fact, a reflux period of approximately 20 hours with 0.03 normal acid is needed to hydrolyse the dialkanolamide completely. The effect was investigated of increasing the strength of sulphuric acid up to 0.1 normal during reflux. At the end of the reflux the acid strength was adjusted back to 0.03 normal by the addition of sodium hydroxide. Excess periodic acid was then added and the estimation continued as described previously. Because a 5 to 6 hour reflux with 0.1 normal sulphuric acid is needed to hyrolyse lauric diethanolamide completely to diethanolamine (Table 23), lauric diethanolamide was estimated in the distilled water extractants by adjusting the sample to 0.1 normal with respect to sulphuric acid, refluxing for at least 6 hours, and then adjusting back to 0.03 normal acid strength before determination of diethanolamine by the periodic acid method.

TABLE 22

Experimental conditions in the determination of the diethanolamine by the periodic acid method

Diethanolamine (ppm) in 100ml test solution. (0.03N with respect to sulphuric acid)

Reaction time of diethanolamine with 0.02N periodic acid (minutes)	Added	Found	Recovery %	Titre Difference (sample-blank) (0.01N iodine ml)	Added	Found	Recovery %	Titre Difference (sample-blank) (0.01N iodine ml)	Added	Found	Recovery %	Titre Difference (sample-blank) (0.01N iodine ml)
20	14	13	93	4.9	31	29	94	-	-	-	-	-
30	14	13	93	4.9	31	27	87	10.3	36	34	94	12.9
60	14	13	93	4.9	31	27	87	-	36	34	94	12.9

In this procedure the sample (100ml) containing between 14 and 36ppm diethanolamine (1.4 to 3.6mg) was reacted for various periods of time, between 20 and 60 minutes, with excess 0.01 molar periodic acid in 0.03 normal sulphuric acid medium. To this solution was added excess 0.02 normal sodium arsenite and sodium bicarbonate. Unused arsenite was then back titrated with 0.01N iodine solution using potentiometric titration using a platinum foil indicating electrode — calomel reference electrode. These results show that it is possible to determine diethanolamine amounts down to about 3ppm in the 100ml of test solution, with a recovery of about 90% or higher of the amount added.

TABLE 23

Investigation of hydrolysis conditions required for the conversion
of lauric diethanolamide*to diethanolamine

Sulphuric acid reflux time, hours	Recovery (% of added amount of lauric diethanolamide)**		
	Concentration of sulphuric acid present during hydrolysis of lauric diethanolamide		
	0.03 normal	0.05 normal	0.10 normal
1	29	32	42
2	38	49	64
3	52	60	80
4	–	–	93
5	–	79	100
6	70	–	100
9	82	–	–
16	96	–	–

*   Using commercial lauric diethanolamide which had been twice recrystallised
from methanol (assumed to be 100% lauric diethanolamide for the purpose of
calculating results).

** 12mg recrystallised lauric diethanolamide used in each experiment.

Composition of Original Lauric Diethanolamide

Component	% w/w
$C_{11}H_{23}CON(CH_2CH_2OH)_2$	80.6
$HN\begin{cases} CH_2CH_2OOCC_{11}H_{23} \\ CH_2CH_2OH \end{cases}$	7.1
$C_{11}H_{23}CON\begin{cases} CH_2CH_2OOCC_{11}H_{23} \\ CH_2CH_2OH \end{cases}$	4.7
$C_{11}H_{23}CON(CH_2CH_2OOCC_{11}H_{23})_2$	0.0
Free diethanolamine	0.0
Free fatty acid	0.0
Water	7.6

The results in Table 24 confirm that lauric diethanolamide is indeed hydrolysed by contact with distilled water for 10 days at 60°C. To estimate free diethanolamine, one portion of the extractant was analysed directly by the periodic acid procedure. The other portion of extractant was refluxed with 0.1 normal sulphuric acid for 6 hours to hydrolyse the diakanolamide completely to diethanolamine, which was then analysed by the periodic acid method (i.e. total undegraded lauric diethanolamide plus degraded dialkanolamide. About 50% of the amount of lauric diethanolamide originally added was hydrolysed by heating in water for 10 days at 60°C.

TABLE 24

Hydrolysis of lauric diethanolamide in distilled

water during 10 days at 60°C

Lauric diethanol-amide (g/100ml test solution)				% of original Lauric diethanolamide addition	
Added	Found			Hydrolysed during extraction test	Not hydrolysed during extraction test
Total 'A'	Total 'B'	Degraded 'C'	Undegraded ('B'-'C')	$\dfrac{'C'}{'A'}$ 100	$\dfrac{('B'-'C')}{'A'}$ 100
0.0008	0.0010	-	-	-	-
0.0017	0.0015	-	-	-	-
	0.0017				
0.0020	0.0022				
	0.0022				
0.0040	0.0040	0.0017	0.0023	42.5	47.5

Determination of lauric diethanolamide and diethanolamine in the aqueous 5% sodium carbonate extractant

As lauric diethanolamide is extensively hydrolysed to diethanolamine by distilled water (i.e. heating for 10 days at 60°C) it would be expected that even more extensive hydrolysis of the additive might occur under the alkaline conditions prevailing in the case of the 5% w/v sodium carbonate extractant. The results in Table 25 show that lauric diethanolamide is almost completely hydrolysed to diethanolamine and fatty acid in aqueous sodium carbonate when heated to 60°C for 10 days.

Determination of lauric diethanolamide and diethanolamine w/v aqueous ethyl alcohol extractant

In the 50% w/v aqueous ethyl alcohol extractant, lauric diethanolamide is not completely hydrolysed to diethanolamine when refluxed in the presence of 0.1 normal sulphuric acid for periods up to 8 hours (i.e. low total recoveries obtained).

The results in Table 26 show that the low lauric diethanolamide recoveries must be due to a slowing down in the rate of hydrolysis of lauric diethanolamide to diethanolamine, brought about by the presence of ethyl alcohol during the preliminary reflux with 0.1 normal sulphuric acid.

Experiments on synthetic solutions of lauric diethanolamide in the 50% w/v ethyl alcohol aqueous extractant showed (Table 27) (horizontal columns 1-5) that in the absence of ethyl alcohol a recovery of between 100% and 120% of the added amount of lauric diethanolamide is obtained by the periodic acid method following hydrolysis with either 0.1 normal or 1 normal sulphuric acid for 6 to 8 hours. However, in the presence of ethyl alcohol, the lauric diethanolamide recoveries obtained following hydrolysis with 0.1 normal sulphuric acid (horizontal column 6) are only about two-thirds of the expected value, but when the acid strength during hydrolysis is increased to 1 normal a quantitative lauric diethanolamide recovery is obtained (horizontal columns 7-8). Thus, the low lauric diethanolamide recoveries observed earlier can be overcome by increasing the sulphuric acid strength during hydrolysis from 0.1 to 1.0 normal.

TABLE 25

Hydrolysis of lauric diethanolamide occurring in

5% sodium carbonate during 10 days at $60^{o}C$

Lauric diethanolamide grammes added to 200ml 5% sodium carbonate				% of original lauric diethanolamide addition	
Added		Found		Hydrolysed during extraction test	Not hydrolysed during extraction test
Total 'A'	Total 'B'	Degraded 'C'	Undegraded ('B'-'C')	$\frac{'C'}{'A'}$ 100	$\frac{('B'-'C')}{'A'}$ 100
) 0.0042	0.0042	Nil	105	Nil	
0.0040)					Nil
) 0.0042	0.0042	Nil	105	Nil	

Determination of lauric diethanolamide and hydrolysis products in the 5% w/v aqueous citric acid extractant

The periodic acid method cannot be applied directly to the determination of diethanolamine in the 5% citric extractant due to the fact that citric acid itself reacts with periodic acid and interferes in the analysis. It is, therefore, necessary to devise a method for removing citric acid from this extractant prior to the determination of diethanolamine. By adding a slight excess of barium carbonate to the extractant, citrate ions are precipitated as barium citrate, and the insoluble salt then removed from the solution by centriguging. However, it was found that the clear aqueous phase recovered by this procedure still contained sufficient citrate ions to interfere in the periodic acid method (due, presumably, to the presence of dissolved barium citrate, which is slightly soluble in water). To remove the last trace of barium citrate from the extractant, it was passed down a column of Amberlite I.R.A. 400 ion exchange resin (in the chloride form).

TABLE 26

Determination of Diethanolamine in 50% w/v ethyl alcohol :

water extractant

Reaction time with periodic acid minutes	Concentration of diethanolamine in 100ml test solution ppm	Volume of water added before periodic acid addition ml	Volume of 0.03N sulphuric acid added before periodic acid addition ml	Volume of water added immediately prior to iodine back titration ml	Diethanolamine recovery %
30	15-40	0	0	0	94-104
15-60	15	0	0	100	96-104
30	40	100	0	0	91-99
30	40	0	100	0	48*-95

Method of Analysis:

100ml 50% w/v ethanol : water extractant adjusted to 0.03 normal with respect to sulphuric acid, added 15ml 0.01 molar periodic acid and left to react for 30 minutes. Added 30ml saturated sodium bicarbonate and 25ml 0.02N normal sodium arsenite and left 10 minutes. Added 2ml 15% potassium iodide and 10g solid sodium bicarbonate and back titrated arsenite with standard 0.01 normal iodine.

* Low results due to the presence of too much acid in the reaction mixture during reaction of excess periodic acid with sodium arsenite.

TABLE 27

Hydrolysis of lauric diethanolamide by sulphuric acid in distilled water and in ethyl alcohol:water media (refluxed for 6 to 8 hours)

The requirement for a higher concentration of acid for complete hydrolysis in the presence of alcohol (Expt. No. 6)

No.	Dilution of extraction liquid with distilled water	Concentration of lauric diethanolamide in original 200 ml extraction liquid (ppm)	Volume of diluted extraction liquid used for determination of lauric diethanolamide (ml)	Concentration of ethyl alcohol in diluted extraction liquid during reflux with sulphuric acid (% w/v)	Concentration of sulphuric acid in diluted extraction liquid during reflux (Normality)	Volume of distilled water added to extraction liquid immediately prior to iodine back titration (ml)	Recovery of added lauric diethanolamide (%)
1	200 ml distilled water extractant diluted to 250 ml	8	100a	0	0.1	0	120
2	- ditto -	20	100a	0	0.1	0	110
3	- ditto -	17	100a	0	0.1	100	99
4	- ditto -	69	100a	0	1.0	100	101
5	200 ml distilled water extractant diluted to 500 ml	69	200b	0	1.0	200	100
6	200 ml ethyl alcohol: water extractant diluted to 250 ml	40	100a	40	0.1	100	62, 66
7	- ditto - c	69	100a	40	1.0	100	102, 99
8	200 ml ethyl alcohol: water extractant diluted to 500 ml	69	200b	20	1.0	200	101

a   100 ml Extraction liquid adjusted to 0.1 normal or 1.0 normal with sulphuric acid and refluxed for 6 to 8 hours to hydrolyse lauric diethanolamide to diethanolamine. Solution adjusted back to 0.03N with respect to sulphuric acid by addition of sodium hydroxide. Added 15 ml 0.01 molar periodic acid and left for 30 minutes. Added 30 ml saturated sodium bicarbonate and 25 ml 0.02 normal sodium arsenite and left 10 min. Added 2 ml of 18% potassium iodide, 10 g solid sodium bicarbonate, and back titrated excess arsenite and 0.01 normal iodine.

b   As above but double quantities were used of periodic acid and all other subsequently added reagents.

c   When 200 ml 50% w/v ethyl alcohol: water extractant is diluted to 250 ml with water, then the final mixture contains 40% w/v ethyl alcohol (see horizontal column 7 in Table 27). A 100 ml portion of this solution is adjusted to 1 normal with respect to sulphuric acid, refluxed to hydrolyse Ethylan MLD, and then adjusted back to 0.03 normal acid strength by addition of sodium hydroxide prior to determination of diethanolamine. Owing to its high alcohol content, this solution precipitates out some sodium sulphate which causes difficulties in the subsequent analysis for diethanolamine. To overcome this, the original 200 ml 50% w/v ethyl alcohol: water extractant is diluted to 500 ml with water (i.e. final solution contains 20% w/v ethyl alcohol, see horizontal column 8 in Table 27) A 200 ml portion of this adjusted to 1 normal with respect to sulphuric acid and treated as described above. This solution, upon addition to sodium hydroxide, does not precipitate out sodium sulphate and can be satisfactorily analysed for its diethanolamine content.

Citrate ions remained on the ion-exchange column and diethanolamine passed through with the column effluent:-

Resin Cl + Ba citrate → Resin citrate + Ba chloride

Blank estimations by the periodic acid method carried out on the 5% citric acid extractant following the barium carbonate precipitation and ion-exchange chromatographic separations described above showed that these procedures had completely removed citrate ions from the extractant liquid.

Table 28 shows the results obtained in applying the citrate removal procedure described above to a synthetic solution of diethanolamine (70ppm w/v) in the 5% citric acid extractant. A recovery of 97% of the added amount of diethanolamine was obtained in the first 500ml of the ion-exchange column effluent, proving that the method is quantitative.

In a further experiment a synthetic solution of lauric diethanolamine (40ppm w/v) in the 5% citric acid extractant was heated for 10 days at $60^{\circ}C$) during which time it was considered likely that citric acid would completely hydrolyse lauric diethanolamide to diethanolamine. The citric acid removal procedure was then applied to the extractant and diethanolamine determined in the column effluent by the periodic acid method. The amount of diethanolamine obtained was that expected, assuming lauric diethanolamide had completely hydrolysed to diethanolamine during the extraction test. Thus, in determining total lauric diethanolamide plus hydrolysed lauric diethanolamide in the 5% citric acid extractant, it is unnecessary to apply the preliminary reflux with 0.1 normal sulphuric acid prior to analysis by the periodic acid method.

Determination of lauric diethanolamide in the liquid paraffin extractant

Although complete or partial hydrolysis of lauric diethanolamide to diethanolamine occurs with the four aqueous extractants no such hydrolysis was expected in the case of a solution of lauric diethanolamide in the liquid paraffin extractant.

Table 29 gives the results obtained in checks for the presence of diethanolamine in synthetic liquid paraffin solutions of lauric diethanolamide after it had been heated for 10 days at $60^{\circ}C$. At the end of the extraction test the solution (20ppm w/v lauric diethanolamide) was diluted with cyclohexane and divided into two portions for determination of diethanolamine and undegraded lauric diethanolamide.

Diethanolamine is water-soluble and can be determined by applying the periodic acid method to a water extract of the liquid paraffin/cyclohexane mixture. A small amount of diethanolamine was found in the liquid paraffin extractant (less than 20% of the 20ppm w/v of lauric diethanolamide present in the liquid paraffin before the extraction test, see Table 29; some of which was present as an impurity in the original batch of lauric diethanolamide used in this work.

To determine lauric diethanolamide, a further portion of the cyclohexane solution of liquid paraffin was refluxed with 0.5 normal sulphuric acid until complete hydrolysis to diethanolamine had occurred. Under these conditions, a twenty-four hour reflux period was needed to hydrolyse lauric diethanolamide completely. Determination of total diethanolamine in the water extract by the periodic acid method (Table 29) showed that the lauric diethanolamide recovery was reasonably near to the theoretical value.

Detailed procedures are given below for the determination of lauric diethanolamide

TABLE 28

Determination of lauric diethanolamide and diethanolamine
in the 5% w/v aqueous citric acid extractant

Weight (g) of diethanolamine found in various ion exchange column fractions				Total weight (g) diethanolamine		Diethanolamine recovery %
Fraction 1 (250ml)	Fraction 2 (100ml)	Fraction 3 (100ml)	Fraction 4 (100ml)	Found	Added	
Synthetic solution of diethanolamine (0.0140g) in 5% citric acid (200ml)						
0.0134	0.0001	<0.0001	<0.0001	0.0135	0.0140	97
Synthetic solution of lauric diethanolamide (0.0080g)* in 5% citric acid, (200ml heated under B.P.F. test conditions, i.e. 10 days at 60°C) before application of barium carbonate precipitation and ion-exchange procedures.						
0.0025	0.0004	< 0.0001	–	0.0029	0.0029*	100

* The weight of lauric diethanolamide taken (0.0080g) would, upon complete hydrolysis yield 0.0029g diethanolamine. The fact that this weight of diethanolamine was obtained in the column effluent indicated that lauric diethanolamide is completely hydrolysed by 5% citric acid during 10 days at 60°C, i.e. the sulphuric acid hydrolysis step can be omitted in the analysis.

and   diethanolamine in amounts down to 3ppm in the aqueous extractants and in liquid paraffin recommended by the British Plastics Federation.

METHOD

Apparatus

Apparatus required for carrying out extractability test –

Calibrated glassware – Pipettes 100, 50, 25 ml; burettes 50 ml ; volumetric flasks 250, 500 ml.

Miscellaneous glassware – Conical flasks 500, 250 ml ; separating funnels 500 ml.

Apparatus for ion-exchange chromatography of 5% citric acid extractant – Column (length 18in, internal diameter $\frac{7}{8}$ in) fitted at lower end with a No. 2 porosity sinter and a tap.

Centrifuge – M.S.E. Super Medium obtainable from M.S.E. Scientifice Limited (or

TABLE 29

Determination of lauric diethanolamide* and diethanolamine in the liquid paraffin extractant after 10 days at 60°C

| Added | Lauric diethanolamide Found | | | % of original lauric diethanolamide addition | |
| | Total* 'B' | Diethanolamine** 'C' | Undegraded 'B'-'C' | As diethanolamine $\frac{'C'}{'A'}$ 100 | As lauric diethanolamide $\frac{('B'-'C')}{'A'}$ 100 |
Total 'A'					
0.0080	0.0096	0.0015	0.0081	19	101
0.0080	0.0097	0.0013	0.0084	16	105

* Using commercial lauric diethanolamide (which had not been recrystallised from methanol). Lauric diethanolamide assumed for the purpose of calculating results to be 100% pure lauric diethanolamide, although it is evident from these results that this assumption is not quite correct (total lauric diethanolamide recovery some 20% higher than expected).

** Determined as diethanolamine, calculated as lauric diethanolamide.

equivalent instrument).

REAGENTS

Periodic acid - 0.01 molar, weigh out 2.28g of periodic acid (HIO 2H 0) to four decimal places, and dissolve in approximately 100ml of distilled water. Transfer quantitatively to a 1 litre standard volumetric flask, dilute to the mark and mix thoroughly.

Sodium arsenite 0.02N - Dissolve 0.8g of sodium hydroxide Analar and 1.0g of arsenious oxide Analar in the minimum quantity of distilled water, warm in the beaker to obtain complete solution. Transfer quantitatively to a 1 litre standard volumetric flask and add 2.0g of solid bicarbonate Analar, swirl the flask until the solid is completely dissolved, dilute to the mark and mix thoroughly.

Iodine solution 0.01N - Prepared from 0.1N iodine

Dilute 100ml of this solution to 1 litre with distilled water.

Potassium iodide 15% aqueous. Dissolve 15g of potassium iodide Analar in 100ml of water.

Sodium bicarbonate - saturated aqueous.

Sodium bicarbonate - Analar - solid.

Sodium hydroxide - 5N aqueous. Dissolve 200g of sodium hydroxide Analar in water and dilute to 1 litre. Accurately standardise to three places of decimals.

Sodium hydroxide - N aqueous. Accurately standardised.

Sulphuric acid - 10N aqueous. Dilute 70ml concentrated sulphuric acid Analar (S.G. 1.84) to 250ml with distilled water. Accurately standardise to three places of decimals.

Sulphuric acid - 5N aqueous. Accurately standardised.

Sulphuric acid - 0.03N aqueous. Accurately standardised.

Hydrochloric acid 1N - Accurately standardised.

Ethanol - absolute.

Cyclohexane - re-distil cyclohexane and discard the first and last 10% of the distillate.

Methyl Orange indicator - 0.02% aqueous.

Barium carbonate - solid Analar.

Ion exchange resin - Amberlite IRA 400-Cℓ (available from British Drug Houses Limited, Poole, Dorset).

Starch 1% - aqueous.

PROCEDURE

Transfer of liquids from extraction tubes

(a) Take the tube used in the extractability test containing 200ml extraction
liquid, and warm to 60°C in a water bath for a few minutes. Shake the tube to
mix thoroughly and disperse any insolubles. Transfer the warm liquid from the
extraction tube into a 250ml standard volumetric flask. Rinse out the
extraction tube with three separate 10ml portions of hot ethanol (to dissolve any
deposited solid adhering to the walls of the tube) and transfer these washings
to the volumetric flasks. Allow the solution to cool to room temperature, make
up to 250ml with distilled water and mix thoroughly.

Analysis of distilled water extractant

(b) Determination of the free diethanolamine content of the distilled water
extractant. Pipette 100ml of the diluted extraction liquid referred to in
Section (a) into a 250ml conical flask. Add 6.5ml of 0.5N standardised
sulphuric acid solution (i.e. sufficient acid to adjust the solution to
approximately 0.03N with respect to sulphuric acid). Into a second flask (blank)
pipette 100ml of 0.03N aqueous sulphuric acid.

(c) Into the sample and blank flasks pipette 15ml of 0.01 molar periodic acid
solution and leave to react for 30 1 minutes. Immediately add 30ml of saturated
sodium bicarbonate solution and 25ml of 0.02N sodium arsenite solution. Leave
to react for 10±1 minutes. Add 2ml of 15% potassium iodide solution and 10g
of solid sodium bicarbonate, swirl to dissolve the sodium bicarbonate and add a
few drops of starch indicator solution. Titrate the solution with 0.01N iodine
to the blue end-point (blue colour should persist for at least two minutes).
Record the sample and blank iodine titrations.

An alternative method of end-point detection is by means of a potentiometric
titration procedure using either manual methods or an automatic titrimeter (see
Note 1 and Figure 58).

(d) Calculate the weight of free diethanolamine present in the whole 250ml of
test solution.

(e) Determination of lauric diethanolamide in the distilled water extractant.
Pipette a further 100ml portion of the 250ml of extractant referred to in Section
(a) into a 250ml conical flask. Into a 250ml flask blank) pipette 100ml of
0.03N sulphuric acid. Pipette accurately 1ml of standardised 10N sulphuric acid
solution into the sample flask and attach a vertical condenser. Reflux the
sample solution for 8 hours on a hot plate to hydrolyse diethanolamide to
diethanolamine. At the end of this period allow to cool, and rinse down the
condenser with sufficient distilled water to make the volume up to 120ml.   To
this flask add accurately 6.2ml standardised N sodium hydroxide solution (i.e.
sufficient alkali to make the solution about 0.03N with respect to sulphuric
acid). Proceed as described in Section (c).

(f) Calculate the weight of lauric diethanolamide present in the whole 250ml
of test solution.

Analysis of 5% sodium carbonate extractant

(g) Determination of free diethanolamine content of the sodium carbonate extractant.
Transfer the 5% aqueous sodium carbonate extractant from the extraction tube to a
250ml volumetric flask with distilled water, as described in Section (a).

Pipette 25ml of this solution into a 100ml conical flask, add a few drops of methyl orange indicator solution, and titrate with standardised normal hydrochloric acid solution to the pink coloured end-point. Calculate the normality of the sodium carbonate solution (1 litre N hydrochloric acid is equivalent to 1 litre N sodium carbonate solution :- 53g per litre, at the methyl orange end-point).

(h) Pipette 100ml of the extraction liquid into a 250ml conical flask and add, from a graduated pipette, a calculated volume of accurately standardised 10N sulphuric acid (sufficient to neutralise the sodium carbonate present and make the final volume of solution 0.03N with respect to sulphuric acid - see Section (g)). Into a second (blank) flask, pipette 100ml 0.03N sulphuric acid. Proceed as described in Section (c).

Calculate the weight of diethanolamine present in the whole 250ml of test solution.

(i) Determination of lauric diethanolamide in 5% sodium carbonate extractant. Pipette 100ml of the extraction liquid into a 250ml conical flask and add, from a graduated pipette, a calculated volume of accurately standardised 10N sulphuric acid sufficient to neutralise the sodium carbonate present and make the final volume of solution 0.1N with respect to sulphuric acid (see Section (g)). Into a second (blank) flask pipette 100ml 0.03N sulphuric acid. Attach a condenser to the sample flask and reflux for 8 hours to hydrolyse lauric diethanolamide to diethanolamine. Allow the flask to cool, and rinse down the condenser with sufficient distilled water to make the volume up to 120ml. To this flask add accurately 6.2ml standardised N sodium hydroxide solution (i.e. sufficient alkali to make the solution about 0.03N with respect to sulphuric acid). Proceed as described in Section (c). Calculate the weight of lauric diethanolamide in the whole 250ml of test solution.

Analysis of liquid paraffin extractant

(j) Transference of liquid paraffin from extraction tube. At the end of the B.P.F. extraction test, remove the extraction tube from the constant temperature bath, mix the contents well, and clean the outside of the tube thoroughly with a cloth. With a pair of clean tongs remove the sample from the tube and allow the liquid paraffin adhering to the sample to drain back into the tube. Transfer the extractant to a 500ml standard volumetric rlask, rinsing out the extraction tube with a 5 × 60ml portion of warm cyclohexane, and add these washings to the contents of the 500ml flask. Allow the solution to cool to room temperature, dilute to the mark with cyclohexane and mix thoroughly.

(k) Determination of the free diethanolamine content of the liquid paraffin extractant. Measure 200ml of the 500ml of cyclohexane solution of liquid paraffin into a 500ml separating funnel, wash this solution with a 4 × 50ml portion of 0.03N sulphuric acid and run these washings into a 500ml conical flask. Into a second (blank) flask run 200ml 0.03N sulphuric acid.

(1) Into the sample and blank flasks run 30ml of 0.01 molar periodic acid and leave to react for 30 ± 1 minutes. Immediately add 60ml of saturated sodium bicarbonate solution and 50ml of 0.02N sodium arsenite solution. Leave to react for 10 ± 1 minutes. Add 4ml of 15% potassium iodide solution and 20g solid sodium bicarbonate, swirl to dissolve and add a few drops of starch indicator solution. Titrate the solution with 0.01N iodine to the blue end-point (blue colour should persist for at least two minutes). Record the sample and blank iodine titrations.

(m) Calculate the weight of free diethanolamine present in the whole 500ml of cyclohexane test solution.

(n) Determination of lauric diethanolamide in the liquid paraffin extractant.
Measure a further 200ml portion of the 500ml of cyclohexane solution of liquid
paraffin into a 500ml conical flask and accurately pipette in 12ml of 0.5N
sulphuric acid solution. Place the flask on a magnetic stirrer/hot plate and
agitate the solution by means of a stirrer bar. Attach a condenser to the flask
and reflux for 24 hours. Allow the solution to cool, wash down the condenser with
a few ml of distilled water, and run the cyclohexane and aqueous phase into a
500ml separating funnel. Carefully rinse the reflux flask with 50ml distilled
water and 20ml cyclohexane, and transfer these washings to the separator funnel.
Wash the organic layer with several 50ml portions of distilled water and run the
water washings in a 250ml conical flask using a total of 200ml of water for the
extractions, i.e. final extract is 0.03N with respect to sulphuric acid. Into a
second (blank) conical flask run 200ml of 0.03N sulphuric acid. Proceed as
described in Section (1). Calculate the weight of lauric diethanolamide present
in the whole 500ml of cyclohexane test solution.

Analysis of 50% w/v ethanol : water extractant

(o) Take the tube used in the extractability test and warm to 60°C in a water
bath for a few minutes. Shake the tube thoroughly, mix and disperse any insolubles.
Transfer the warm liquid from the extraction tube into a 500ml volumetric flask.
Rinse out the tube with three separate 10ml portions of hot ethanol (to dissolve
any deposited diethanolamine adhering to the walls of the tube) and transfer these
washings to the volumetric flask. Allow to cool to room temperature, make up to
500ml with distilled water and mix thoroughly.

(p) Determination of free diethanolamine in 50% w/v ethanol : water extractant.
Measure 200ml of the diluted extractant into a conical flask and accurately
pipette in 13ml standardised 0.5N sulphuric acid from a graduated pipette (i.e.
sufficient acid to adjust the solution to 0.03N with respect to sulphuric acid).
Into a second (blank) flask pipette 200ml 0.03N sulphuri acid. Proceed as
described in Section (1).

It will be observed that, under the above conditions, the 20g solid sodium
bicarbonate added immediately prior to the iodine titration does not always
completely dissolve (due to the presence of a high concentration of ethyl alcohol).
Solubilise the sodium bicarbonate at this stage of the analysis by adding 100ml
distilled water to the sample and the blank solutions immediately prior to the
iodine titration.

Calculate the weight of free diethanolamine present in the whole 500ml of test
solution.

(q) Determination of lauric diethanolamide in 50% w/v ethanol : water extractant.
Accurately measure 200ml of the 500ml extractant referred to in Section (o) into
a 500ml conical flask. Into another (blank) flask measure 200ml of 0.03N sulphuric
acid. Into the sample flask accurately pipette 22.2ml of standardised 10N
sulphuric acid (i.e. diluted solution is 1.0N with respect to sulphuric acid
- see Note 2). Attach a condenser to the flask and reflux for 8 hours to hydrolyse
lauric diethanolamide to diethanolamine. Allow the flask to cool, and rinse down
the condenser with a few ml of distilled water. To the sample solution add a few
drops of methyl orange indicator solution, and titrate with standardised 5N
sodium hydroxide solution to the yellow-coloured end-point (the theoretical
titration of 5.00N sodium hydroxide is 44.4ml). Then add accurately, by pipette,
sufficient standardised 10N sulphuric acid to convert to the solution to 0.03N
with respect to sulphuric acid (the theoretical addition of 10.0N sulphuric acid
is 0.8ml). Proceed as described in Section (1). If the 20g addition of sodium

bicarbonate made immediately before the iodine titration of the sample does not completely dissolve (due to the presence of a high concen tration of ethanol), add 100ml distilled water to solubilise the sodium bicarbonate before carrying out the iodine titration.

Calculate the weight of lauric diethanolamide present in the whole 500ml of test solution.

Analysis of 5% w/v citric acid extractant (Note 3)

(r) Transfer the 5% aqueous citric acid extractant from the extraction tube into a 250ml volumetric flask as described in section (a).

Only free diethanolamine need be determined in this extractant as it has been shown that lauric diethanolamide is completely hydrolysed in this medium to diethanolamine during the course of 10-day extractability test at 60°C (Note 4).

(s) Removal of major proportion of citric acid from extractant. Into a 250ml centrifuge bottle, accurately pipette a 120ml portion of the 250ml citric acid extractant referred to in Section (r). Into a second (blank) 250ml centrifuge bottle, measure 100ml 5% citric acid extractant which has not been in contact with the plastic sample. To each bottle add 8 ± 0.1g (i.e. 20% to 30% excess) of solid barium carbonate. Stir for one hour to enable the barium carbonate to convert citric acid into insoluble barium citrate.

Centrifuge the bottles for one hour at 2,500 rev/min on an M.S.E. Super Medium Centrifuge (or equivalent) to separate an upper clear phase from the settled barium carbonate/bsrium citrate layer. Remove the bottles from the centrifuge and carefully pipette off as much as possible of the clear upper phases without disturbing the settled solid phase. Measure the volume of clear liquid recovered (it should be possible to recover 90 to 100ml of the undiluted citric acid extractant liquid at this stage of the analysis) and filter the clear phase into two 250ml separatory funnels. Wash through the filter papers into the separatory funnels with 50ml distilled water.

(t) Removal of the last trace of citric acid from extractant by ion exchange chromatography (see Note 3). Prepare an ion exchange column of Amberlite IRA 400 Cl as follows:- Slurry 130g Amberlite IRA 400 Cl resin in 200ml distilled water and completely transfer it into an 18" chromatographic column (7/18" diameter) fitted at the lower end with a No.2 porpsity sintered disc and stopcock. Allow the column to drain until the water level is just above the level of the re sin.

To the top of the ion exchange column, connect a separatory funnel containing the centrifugate referred to in Section(s). To the lower end of the column connect a one-litre conical flask. Run the liquid into the column at a rate of 2 to 3ml per minute, always keeping the liquid level just above the level of the resin in the column. When the sample has run through the column, run through distilled water until a total volume of 400ml of effluent has been collected. To the sample extract flask (A) and the citric acid blank flask (B) (each containing 400ml of effluent) add accurately by pipette 1.3ml of 10N sulphuric acid (i.e. sufficient acid to convert the solution to 0.03N with respect to sulphuric acid). To a third (distilled water blank) flask (C), add 400ml of 0.03N sulphuric acid.

(u) Determination of diethanolamine. To the three flasks (A, B and C) add 60ml 0.01 molar periodic acid and allow the solution to react for 30 ± 1 minute. Then add 120ml of saturated sodium bicarbonate solution and 100ml 0.02N sodium arsenite and allow to react for 10 ± 1 minutes. Add 8ml 15% potassium iodide and 40g solid sodium bicarbonate. Swirl to dissolve the sodium bicarbonate and add a few drops of starch indicator. Titrate the solutions with 0.01N iodine solution to the blue end-point (blue colour should persist for at least two minutes).

The iodine titration obtained with flask (B) should be identical to the blank titration obtained with flask (C). This confirm that citric acid has been completely removed from the citric acid blank solution by barium carbonate treatment and ion-exchange chromatography. From the iodine titrations obtained with the sample flask (A) and the reagent blank flask (C) claculate the weight of diethanolamine present in the whole 250ml of original test solution (Section (r)).

CALCULATION

Determination of free diethanolamine in extraction liquid

Weight (g) of diethanolamine present in volume of extraction liquid in contact with plastic

$$= \frac{(T_s - T_B) \times f \times 105.1 \times V_2}{10^3 \times 4 \times V_1} = A \text{ g diethanolamine}$$

where V_2 = volume (ml) of extraction liquid in contact with plastic during extractability test;

V_1 = actual volume (ml) of above extraction liquid represented by portion of sample used in periodic acid analysis;

T_s = back titration (ml) of iodine obtained with sample;

T_B = back titration (ml) of iodine obtained in reagent blank determination; and

f = normality of iodine solution.

Weight (g) of lauric diethanolamide present in volume of extraction liquid in contact with plastic

$$= \frac{(t_s - t_B) \times f \times 105.1 \times V_3}{10^3 \times 4 \times V_4} - A \quad \frac{M}{105.1}$$

where V_3 = volume (ml) of extraction liquid in contact with plastic during extractability test;

V_4 = actual volume (ml) of above extraction liquid represented by portion of sample used in periodic acid analysis;

t_s = back titration (ml) of iodine obtained with sample;

t_B = back titration (ml) of iodine obtained in reagent blank determination;

f = normality of iodine solution.

     A = weight (g) of diethanolamine present in volume of extraction liquid in contact with plastic, (see above); and

     M = molecular weight of lauric diethanolamide (see Note 5).

NOTE 1 Alternative methods for end-point detection in sodium arsenite/iodine titrations

The end-point of the sodium arsenite/iodine titration may be determined potentiometrically and the titration may be carried out using an automatic titrator or a pH meter. The electrode system consists of a glass electrode as reference and a platinum electrode as the measuring electrode. The platinum electrode consists of a 1cm square of platinum foil suspended on the tip of a normal platinum wire electrode.

An excess of iodine in the solution is denoted by a sharp increased in potential of the electrode system, and the point at which this change takes place is the end-point (see Figure 58).

NOTE 2 Difficulty of hydrolysis of lauric diethanolamide in N/10 sulphuric acid

Lauric diethanolamide hydrolyses more slowly in 50% w/v aqueous ethanol than in the other aqueous extractants in the presence of 0.1N sulphuric acid. The acidity of this solution is therefore increased to normal, and the hydrolysis time to 8 hours, in order to bring about quantitative hydrolyses of lauric diethanolamide.

NOTE 3 Interference by citric acid in the periodic acid method for estimation of diethanolamine

Under the conditions of the analysis, citric acid consumes periodic acid and therefore interferes in the determination of diethanolamine. Citric acid is removed from the citric acid and extractant prior to determination of diethanolamine by the following procedure.

To the citric acid extractant is added an excess of barium carbonate. This precipitates off from the clear aqueous phase by centrifuging. Unfortunately, owing to the slight solubility of barium citrate in water, sufficient citrate ions still remain in solution after this procedure to interfere in the periodic acid method. The last traces of citrate ions are removed from the test solution by passing it down a column of Amberlite IRA 400 - Cl resin. Citrate ions are retained in the resin and diethanolamine is quantitatively recovered in the column effluent.

$$R - Cl + Ba\ Citrate = R\ Citrate + Ba\ Chloride$$

Diethanolamine can now be successfully determined in the effluent without interference from citrate ions.

NOTE 4 Hydrolysis of lauric diethanolamide to diethanolamine by the 5% citric acid extractant

It has been shown that 5% citric acid completely hydrolyses lauric diethanolamide to diethanolamine during the extractability test carried out on the plastic under

the conditions of the British Plastics Federation, i.e. 10 days at 60°C. There is
no need, therefore, to determine lauric diethanolamide in this extractant.

NOTE 5 Molecular weight of lauric diethanolamide

For the purpose of calculating results it may be assumed that lauric diethanolamide
is 100% pure lauric diethanolamide ($C_{11}H_{23}CON (CH_2CH_2OH)_2$) which has a molecular
weight of 287. Alternatively, the procedure may be calibrated against a specimen
of the same batch of lauric diethanolamide that was included in the polymer
formulation used from extractability studies. To calibrate the method a known
weight of the lauric diethanolamide is refluxed with N/10 sulphuric acid for 8
hours and the amount of diethanolamine produced is measured by the periodic acid
method.

Some results obtained in applying this procedure to the determination of the
extractability of lauric diethanolamide antistatic agent from a range of plastic
materials are given in Tables 30-32.

Extractability determinations were carried out on 1-2 thou thick low-density
polyethylene film, containing 0.03% lauric diethanolamide and 0.1% Aerosil
(silica).

Following the conditions prescribed by the B.P.F. for polymer sections of less
than 0.02 inch thickness, a volume of film up to 10ml was kept in contact with
200ml of each extractant for 10 days at 60°C. The results of these tests are
given in Table 30.

The data in Table 30 indicate that, after it had migrated from the polyethylene
film, lauric diethanolamide extensively hydrolysed to diethanolamine, especially
in the case of the 5% sodium carbonate and 5% citric acid extractants. Also,
between 60% and 100% of the original lauric diethanolamide content of the film
migrated from the film into the extraction liquid during ten days' exposure at
60°C.

The effect of carrying out the extraction test at room temperature instead of at
60°C as illustrated in Table 31. The results show that reduction of the
temperature during the extraction test reduces the rate of migration of lauric
diethanolamide from the film into the extraction liquid. The extracted additive,
however, is still completely hydrolysed to diethanolamine , even when the test is
carried out at 20°C.

Extractability tests carried out on injection moulded polystyrene cups with a
nominal wall thickness of 0.02 inch containing 1.5% lauric diethanolamide as an
antistatic additive using the conditions prescribed by the B.P.F. for plastic
specimens of thicknesses greater than 0.02 inch (i.e. each square cm of plastic
in contact with at least 1ml of extraction liquid). Tests were run for 10 days
at 60°C and total undegraded plus degraded lauric diethanolamide (i.e. diethanolamine)
was determined in each extractant and calculated as grammes lauric diethanolamide
extracted per 4000 sq cm of plastic surface.

The results of these tests are given in Table 32. The total lauric diethanolamide
content of the various extraction liquids at the end of the test was between 3
and 13.5 ppm w/v, and maximum extraction occurred in the case of the liquid
paraffin extractant, 5% sodium carbonate and 50% ethanol : water. Extraction tests
were repeated, using liquid paraffin and 5% sodium carbonate on samples of
polystyrenes containing 1.5% lauric diethanolamide and 2.0% lauric diethanolamide
(Table 33).

TABLE 30

Extractability of Lauric Diethanolamide from 'CARLONA' 18-020 GB low-densidy Polyethylene by B.P.F. extractants

Extractant	Volume of plastic film contacted with 200 ml extractant ml	Lauric diethanolamide g Extracted 100 cc film (a)	Diethanolamine g Extracted/100 cc film		Lauric acid g Extracted per 100 cc film		Total determined (calculated as lauric diethanolamide), g extracted per 100 cc film (a) + (b)	Total added concn. of lauric diethanolamide in original unextracted film, g present/ 100 cc film	% of lauric diethanolamide of extraction liquid hydrolysed to diethanolamine at end of 10 days at 60°C (b) x 100 / (a) + (b)
			Calculated as lauric diethanolamide (b)	Calculated as diethanolamine		Calculated			
Distilled water	6.8 6.8	0.012 0.012	0.005 0.007	0.002 0.002	0.004 0.005		0.018	0.028	Approx. 30
5% Aqueous sodium carbonate	6.3 6.3	0.000 0.000	0.027 0.028	0.010 0.010	0.019 0.020		0.028	0.028	100
50% Aqueous ethanol	7.7 6.5	0.029 0.009 0.006	0.006 0.013 0.017	0.002 0.005 0.006	0.004 0.009 0.012		0.035 0.023	0.028 0.028	Approx. 70
5% Aqueous citric acid	6.3 7.8	0.000 0.000	0.026 0.023	0.010 0.008	0.019 0.017		0.025	0.028	100
Liquid paraffin	6.2 6.2	0.032 0.035	0.000 0.000	0.000 0.000	0.000 0.000		0.033	0.028	Nil

TABLE 31

Extractability of Lauric Diethanolamide from polyethylene into 5% aqueous sodium carbonate at 20°C and 60°C

Extractability test conditions	Volume of plastic film contacted with 200 ml 5% sodium carbonate, ml	Lauric Diethanolamide g Extracted/ 100 cc film (a)	Diethanolamine g Extracted 100 cc film		Total determined (calculated as lauric diethanolamide (g Extracted per 100 cc film)	Total concentration of lauric diethanolamide in original unextracted film (g present/100 cc film)	% of total original lauric diethanolamide content of film extracted during extraction test
			Calculated as lauric diethanolamide (b)	Calculated as diethanolamine			
10 days at 60°C	6.3	0.000 0.000	0.027 0.028	0.010 0.010	0.028	0.028	100
90 days at 20°C	6.2	0.000 0.000	0.020 0.016	0.007 0.006	0.018	0.028	65

TABLE 32

Extractability of lauric diethanolamide from injection moulded polystyrene cups containing

1.5% diethanolamine ('CARINEX' TGX/TW/AS, SI 18)

	Volume of Extractant, ml	Total surface area of plastic sample (both sides), sq cm	Weight of plastic sample, g	Lauric diethanolamide content of 200ml extraction liquid ppm/w/v	Weight of lauric diethanolamide extracted per 4000 sq cm of plastic surface g		% of diethanolamine content of extraction liquid hydrolysed to diethanolamine at end of 10day period at 60°C*
Distilled water	200	100	2.65	3.0±0.5	0.024±0.004		Approx. 30
	200	100	2.64	5.5±0.5	0.044±0.004	Av.0.034 0.004	
5% Sodium carbonate	200	100	2.68	7.5±0.5	0.060±0.004		100
	200	100	2.67	6.0±0.5	0.048±0.004	Av.0.054 0.004	
50% Ethanol : water	200	100	2.44	4.5±0.5	0.036±0.004		Approx. 70
	200	100	2.61	6.0±0.5	0.048±0.004		
	200	104	2.59	5.1±0.5	0.040±0.004	Av.0.051 0.004	
	200	100	2.65	10.1±0.5	0.081±0.004		
5% citric acid	200	109	3.73	2.9±0.5	0.022±0.004		100
	200	97	2.42	2.9±0.5	0.024±0.004	Av.0.023 0.004	
Liquid paraffin	200	100	2.58	13.5±0.5	0.108±0.004		Nil
	200	100	2.46	13.5±0.5	0.108±0.004	Av.0.108 0.004	

* Based on results in Table 30.

Comparison under Set 1 and Set 2 of results obtained for the 5% sodium carbonate and liquid paraffin extractants in tests on polystyrene containing 1.5% lauric diethanolamide shows that two to three times as much diethanolamine and lauric diethanolamide, respectively, was present in extracts obtained in the second test (Set 2), compared with those obtained in the first test (Set 1). Also, as expected, a perceptibly higher concentration of lauric diethanolamide (or its hydrolysis product) was present in the extracts obtained for polystyrene containing 2.0% lauric diethanolamide compared with polystyrene containing 1.5% lauric diethanolamide.

Finally, the extractability tests in 5% sodium carbonate and liquid paraffin were repeated several months later, on different samples of the polystyrene containing 1.5% and 2.0% lauric diethanolamide (Set 3), and the results obtained were very similar to those shown under Set 2.

The results in Table 33 show that the extractability test procedure can be quite reproducible when carried out on different occasions and on different batches of the plastic with a particular additive formulation (compare Sets 2 and 3). However, it is unexpected to find that the results obtained under Set 1 were appreciably lower than those obtained in either of the other two determinations. Three possible explanations for these variable results are proposed below:-

(a)   The first of the samples quoted in Table 33 (Set 1) may have contained less than the stipulated 1.5% lauric diethanolamide, thereby causing low extractability results.

(b)   The degree of extractability of lauric diethanolamide from the polystyrene may have varied with changes in manufacturing processing conditions over a period of time (almost a year elapsed between the analyses shown under Set 1 and Set 2).

(c)   The degree of extractability of lauric diethanolamide from the polystyrene may change with the time interval between polymer manufacture and carrying out the extractability test. During such intervals the antistatic additive may progressively migrate to the plastic surface, and this, in turn may affect results obtained in subsequent extractability tests.

These considerations emphasise the point that it is inadvisable to rely on the results obtained in a single extractability test on a particular polymer formulation. Extractability tests should be repeated over a period of time on different batches of the polymer made in typical manufacturing conditions. In this way it will become evident whether any of the above factors and possibly others, have an effect on the extent of extractability of an additive from a plastic.

The results quoted in Tables 30 to 33 show that lauric diethanolamide is almost completely extracted from 0.002 inch thick low-density polyethylene film into each of the five B.P.F. extractants during 10 days' exposure at 60°C. Complete additive extraction would not necessarily occur in the case of thicker polyethylene films. Also, it has been shown that most, or all, of the lauric diethanolamide extracted from polyethylene or polystyrene is then hydrolysed to diethanolamine and fatty acid; although, of course, this does not occur in the case of the liquid paraffin extractant.

The B.P.F. liquids are intended to simulate various types of foodstuffs and beverages and it seems likely that the hydrolysis of lauric diethanolamide to diethanolamine, referred to above, could also occur in some foodstuffs. Such hydrolytic decomposition of additives might also occur in the case of other types

TABLE 33

Lauric diethanolamide extractability tests carried out on
various polystyrenes containing 1.5% and 2.0% of the
additive

Set 1 (Analysed 1963)

'CARINEX' TGX/TW/AS polystyrene SI 18,
containing 1.5% lauric diethanolamide

g lauric diethanolamide extracted/4000 sq cm
of plastic

Unhydrolysed lauric diethanolamide	Hydrolysed lauric diethanolamide*
Extractant : 5% sodium carbonate	
Nil	0.05, 0.05 Av. 0.05
Extractant : Liquid paraffin	
0.11, 0.11, Av. 0.11	Nil

Set 2 (Analysed (7.5.64)

'CARINEX' TGX/TW/AS polystyrene, Batch G7 containing 1.5% lauric diethanolamide		Polystyrene SI 25B, containing 2.0% lauric diethanolamide	
g lauric diethanolamide extracted per 4000 sq cm plastic			
Unhydrolysed lauric diethanolamide	Hydrolysed lauric diethanolamide	Unhydrolysed lauric diethanolamide	Hydrolysed lauric diethanolamide
Extractant : 5% sodium carbonate			
Nil	0.15,0.26,Av.0.21	Nil	0.39,0.27,Av.0.33
Extractant : Liquid paraffin			
0.21,0.13,Av.0.17	Nil	0.16,0.19,Av.0.18	Nil

* Determined in extractant as diethanolamine and calculated above as lauric
  diethanolamide (assumed to be pure lauric diethanolamide).

<u>TABLE 33 continued</u>

<u>Set 3 (Analysed 23.7.64)</u>

'CARINEX' TGX/TW/AS polystyrene, Batch G7   Polystyrene SI 25B, containing 2.0%
  containing 1.5% lauric diethanolamide   lauric diethanolamide

g lauric diethanolamide extracted per 4000 sq cm plastic

Unhydrolysed lauric diethanolamide	Hydrolysed lauric diethanolamide	Unhydrolysed lauric diethanolamide	Hydrolysed lauric diethanolamide
	Extractant : 5% sodium carbonate		
Nil	0.17,0.21,Av.0.19	Nil	0.32,0.28,Av.0.30
	Extractant : Liquid paraffin		
0.15,0.16,Av.0.15	Nil	0.21,0.17,Av.0.19	Nil

of polymer additives (e.g. those containing ester and substituted amide groups).
In the case of lauric diethanolamide it is obvious that the toxicity of its two
hydrolysis products should be taken into account just as much as the toxicity of
the additive itself.

The results in Table 31 show that hydrolysis of lauric diethanolamide occurs even
when the extraction test is run at room temperature instead of 60°C (tests run
using the 5% sodium carbonate extractant). Thus, if foodstuffs and beverages are
packaged in plastic containers, then even at room temperature, the food or
beverage could pick up diethanolamine and fatty acid produced by hydrolysis of
migrated lauric diethanolamide.

It has also been shown that lauric diethanolamide is hydrolysed fairly rapidly by
human gastric juice at body temperature. Thus, it seems that even if lauric
diethanolamide which has been extracted from a plastic into a foodstuff is not
hydrolysed during storage in the container, it could still be hydrolysed
following ingestion.

Use of infra-red spectroscopy for detection of additive breakdown.
Dilauryl thiodipropionate does not absorb in the ultra-violet region of the spectrum
but does absorb strongly in the infra-red region. The carbonyl absorptopn occurring
at 5.72 microns is a useful wavelength for estimating dilauryl thiodipropionate.
Infra-red spectroscopy cannot, of course, be applied directly to aqueous solutions,
and this necessitates a preliminary extraction of the dilauryl thiodipropionate from
the aqueous extractants with a low-boiling immiscible organic solvent. As discussed
earlier infra-red spectroscopy can be applied to the direct determination of some
types of additives in the liquid paraffin or hexane extractant, although usually
with poor sensitivity, e.g. smallest amount of dilauryl thiodipropionate which can
be detected in these liquids is about 50 to 100ppm. The solvent extraction step
also provides a concentration factor in the analysis which is essential in order to
achieve the necessary analytical sensitivity of down to 10 to 15ppm additive in the
original extraction liquid.

An additional advantage of the infra-red technique is that by comparing the infra-

red spectrum of the solvent extracts of the extraction liquids with that of an
authentic specimen of the dilauryl thiodipropionate it is possible to detect whether
any degradation has occurred, and also to derive information regarding the nature and
degree of such additive degradation.

In addition to dilauryl thiodipropionate, polymers used for extractability tests
might contain other additives which could interfere in an infra-red spectroscopic
method of analysis and these would be present together with dilauryl thiodipropionate
in the extraction liquids. Dilauryl thiodipropionate contains about 6.2% of sulphur.
A Schoniger oxygen flask combustion method is described below for determining sulphur
in the low-boiling organic solvent extract obtained by extraction of the B.P.F.
liquids, and this offers an alternative method for determining dilauryl thiodipropionate in the extractants in those cases where interference is expected in the
infra-red method of analysis.

If good agreement is found between analyses obtained by the oxygen flask combustion
and the infra-red spectroscopic, it can be concluded that true estimates are being
obtained of the dilauryl thiodipropionate content of the extractants.

Based on these principles details are given below of a practical determination of
the extractability of dilauryl thiodipropionate from polypropylene film.

It is always advisable when developing methods of extractant analysis to perform
preliminary experiments on synthetic solutions of known composition of the additive
in the extractant liquids.

Synthetic solutions of dilauryl thiodipropionate were prepared in the four aqueous
and alcoholic extractants. The dilauryl thiodipropionate was added to 700ml of
each of the extractants at the 16 and the 75ppm level as a solution on 5ml methyl
alcohol. These solutions were then heated for 10 days at 60°C in order to simulate
the conditions occurring in an actual polymer extraction test. At the end of this
period, dilauryl thiodipropionate was extracted from the extractants with diethyl
ether preliminary to analysis by the infra-red and oxygen flask procedure.

Diethyl ether extraction of dilauryl thiodipropionate from distilled water, 5% sodium carbonate and 5% citric acid extractants

At the end of the 10-day heating period simulating the extraction test, the 1 litre
extraction tubes were removed from the water bath. The contents whilst still hot
were poured into a 1 litre capacity, upward displacement liquid-liquid extractor.
The interior of the extraction tube was washed with water and diethyl ether which
were transferred to the liquid-liquid extraction thereby avoiding any losses of·
dilauryl thiodipropionate. The contents of the extractor were saturated with solid
sodium chloride to facilitate extraction of dilauryl thiodipropionate during the
subsequent 10 to 15 hours. The ether extract was dried with anhydrous sodium
sulphate and evaporated down prior to making up to volume with ether in a 25ml
volumetric flask.

Diethyl ether extraction of 50% w/v aqueous ethyl alcohol extractant

It is not possible to extract the ethyl alcohol:water extractant directly with
diethyl ether as the two phases are miscible upon mixing. The 700ml ethyl
alcohol:water extractant was distilled down to about 200ml until the distillate
no longer has an odour of ethyl alcohol. The alcohol-free extraction liquid was
then extracted with diethyl ether as described above.

Extraction of dilauryl thiodipropionate from the liquid paraffin extractant

Dilauryl thiodipropionate could not be determined in the liquid paraffin extractant

TABLE 34

Extraction of dilaurylthiodipropionate from liquid paraffin extractant with low-boiling solvents

Volume of liquid paraffin used, ml	Volume of cyclohexane used to dilute liquid paraffin, ml	Original dilauryl thiodipropionate content of liquid paraffin ppm	Solvent extraction cycle used	Recovery of dilauryl thiodipropionate in solvent extract, %	% of original liquid paraffin present in solvent extract
700	300	100	20 hour extraction with anhydrous methanol in liquid–liquid extractor	30	10
700	300	100	10–35 hours extraction with anhydrous ethanol in liquid–liquid extractor	30–35	15–30
100–200	0–100	200–400	Four 20ml extractions with anhydrous methanol	<10	2
100–200	0–100	200–400	Four 20ml extractions with 9:1 (v/v) methanol:water	<10	2
100	0	400	Four 20ml extractions with anhydrous ethanol	20	2
100	0	400	Four 20ml extractions with 9:1 (v/v) ethanol:water	<10	2
100	0*	400	Four 20ml extractions with anhydrous acetone	20	10
100–200	0–100	200–400	Four 20ml extractions with 9:1 (v/v) acetone:water	<10	2

* Liquid paraffin and acetone are completely miscible in presence of cyclohexane.

in amounts less than 100ppm by direct infra-red spectroscopy, nor was it possible
to devise a preliminary solvent extraction procedure to obtain a dilauryl
thiodipropionate concentrate as was achieved in the case of the aqueous extractants.
The results obtained in trial extractions of liquid paraffin with various solvents
(Table 34) indicate that neat or anhydrous (10%) methanol, ethanol or acetone do
not extract more than 35% of the dilauryl thiodipropionate present in the liquid
paraffin extractant, even when the extraction is carried out for extended periods
of up to 35 hours using a liquid-liquid extractor. Moreover, from the results
in Table 34 it can be seen that due to the slight miscibility of liquid paraffin
with these various solvents, the extract would contain appreciable amounts of
liquid paraffin which would reduce the concentration factor achieved in the concentration stage and might interfere in a subsequent analytical procedure.
Consequently adsolvent extraction procedure was not available for obtaining a dilauryl
thiodipropionate concentrate from the liquid paraffin extractant.

The oxygen flask combustion method for determining dilauryl thiodipropionate

Further accurately measured portions of the ether extracts of the extraction liquids
referred to in the next paragraph were reduced in volume to about 2ml. This
solution was then quantitatively transferred in portions to a piece of filter
paper with a dropping pipette. The paper was mounted in a oxygen combustion flask
and combusted over dilute hydrogen peroxide solution. The amount of sulphuric acid
thus produced was estimated by titration with N/100 sodium hydroxide to the
methyl red-methylene blue end-point.

The infra-red spectroscopic method for determination of dilauryl thiodipropionate

Accurately pipetted portions of the ether extract referred to previously were
transferred to small, dry beakers and evaporated to dryness with a nitrogen
stream. The residue was made up to volume with carbon tetrachloride in a 10ml
volumetric flask. Figures 59 (a) and (b) show the infra-red spectra in the 2 to
15 micron region of

(a) synthetic solution of dilauryl thiodipropionate in carbon tetrachloride

(b) dilauryl thiodipropionate found in ether extract of distilled water, 50%
    w/w ethyl alcohol:water, 5% sodium carbonate and 5% citric acid extractants
    after 10 days at 60°C.

Comparison of the infra-red spectrum of dilauryl thiodipropionate (Figure 59 (a))
with those of the ether extracts of the B.P.F. extractants (Figure 59 (b)) shows
that the infra-red spectrum is virtually unchanged by heating dilauryl thiodipropionate for 10 days at 60°C in the various B.P.F. extractants.

To determine quantitatively dilauryl thiodipropionate in the ether extracts of
the various extraction liquids, the infra-red method was calibrated at the 5.72
micron carbonyl absorption against synthetic solutions of pure dilauryl thiodipropionate in carbon tetrachloride.

It Table 35 are shown dilauryl thiodipropionate recoveries obtained by the infra-
red and the oxygen flask methods for synthetic solutions of 16ppm and 75ppm
dilauryl thiodipropionate in the four aqueous extractants. These results show that
by either method of analysis with the exception of the citric acid extractant,
dilauryl thiodipropionate recoveries usually exceed 70% to 80% of the amount
added to the original extraction liquid before the heating period for 10 days at
60°C.

As will be seen in Table 35 dilauryl thiodipropionate recoveries of up to 40%
lower than expected are obtained by the ether-extraction/infra-red method when the

TABLE 35

Recovery of dilauryl thiodipropionate from 700ml aqueous B.P.F.

extractants by ether extraction

Extractant	dilauryl thiodipropionate content of extractant ppm	Recovery of dilauryl thiodipropionate % by ether extraction	
		Determined as sulphur	Determined by infra-red spectroscopy at 5.72 microns
Distilled water	16	80, 83	88
	75	75, 76	82
50% ethyl alcohol water	16	56, 65	69
	75	87	91
5% sodium carbonate	16	73, 82	85
	75	89, 90	92
5% citric acid	16	83, 65	66
	75	39, 49	69

following four extractants have been heated for 10 days at $60^{\circ}C$: distilled water, 1:1 ethanol:water, 5% sodium carbonate, and 5% citric acid. These low recoveries could be due either to (a) incomplete recovery of dilauryl thiodipropionate during ether extraction, or (b) to the occurrence of partial degradation of dilauryl thiodipropionate to another compound brought about by contact with the extraction liquid during the 10 day heating period at $60^{\circ}C$. It was noticed in the case of these three extractants that a white solid was present which was insoluble in the aqueous phase and was not removed by prolonged extraction with ether. Evidently, this solid was not dilauryl thiodipropionate, which is very ether-soluble, but degraded dilauryl thiodipropionate produced during the heating period (the original dilauryl thiodipropionate used in experiments is completely soluble in ether).

In view of the evidence concerning the possible degradation of dilauryl thiodipropionate during the analysis, it is desirable to apply the same treatment to the standard dilauryl thiodipropionate calibration solutions as is applied during the analysis   of plastic extraction liquids of unknown dilauryl thiodipropionate. This would cancel out errors in the analysis caused by partial degradation of dilauryl thiodipropionate. To calibrate the procedure, various standard concentrations of dilauryl thiodipropionate were made up in each of the extractants, which were then heated for 10 days at $60^{\circ}C$. The aqueous extractants were then ether-extracted and the extracts used to calibrate the Schoniger combustion and the infra-red procedures.

The detailed procedures for determining the extractability of dilauryl thiodipropionate from polypropylene film are given below.

Method

Extractability test (British Plastics Federation[1])

Contact the plastic film or sheet with 800ml of each of the four extraction liquids. Use the quantities of plastic and the extraction test conditions as recommended in the Second B.P.F. Toxicity Report[1]. It is convenient to carry out the extraction tests in ground-glass-stoppered tubes of 1 litre capacity. Include in the test polymer-free blank tubes containing 800ml of each extraction liquid.

At the end of the extraction test remove the tubes from the heating bath, shake well and wipe clean. While still hot remove the stopper and remove the plastic. Wash any dilauryl thiodipropionate containing solution from the surface of the plastic into the extraction tube with a jet of warm distilled water (not exceeding 50ml) delivered from a glass wash-bottle.

Extractants - distilled water, 5% sodium carbonate and 5% citric acid

Carefully transfer the hot contents of the extraction tube into a 1 litre capacity liquid-liquid extractor. Wash the interior of the extraction tube with 25ml hot water and two 25ml portions of cold ether, and transfer the washings to the extractor. Proceed as described below.

Extractant - 1:1 ethanol-water

Carefully transfer the hot contents of the extraction tube into a 1 litre, three-necked round-bottomed flask. Wash the interior of the tube with 25ml hot water and two 25ml portions of cold ether and transfer the washings to the 1 litre flask. Connect a separatory funnel containing distilled water, and a horizontally clamped liebeg condenser with suitable adaptor to the flask and distil until the distillate has no odour of ethyl alcohol. Add water to the flask when necessary to keep up the volume to a minimum of 200ml. Ensure that the flask contains between 700 and 800ml of liquid at the end of the distillation. Transfer the hot distillation residue into a 1 litre capacity liquid-liquid extractor. Wash the interior of the flask and the condenser with 25ml hot water and two 25ml portions of cold ether and transfer the washings to the extractor. Proceed as described below.

Ether extraction of extractants

The aqueous ethanol extractant is first distilled to remove alcohol. This extract and the distilled water, 5% sodium carbonate and 5% citric acid extractants are then saturated with sodium chloride and extracted with ether in a liquid-liquid extractor. The ether extract is split into two portions to be used, respectively, for the determination of total sulphur by a Schoniger combustion procedure (Method A) and for the determination of dilauryl thiodipropionate by infra-red spectroscopy at 5.7 microns (Method B).

Ether Extraction Procedure

Reagents

Diethyl ether - shake 4 litres diethyl ether Analar with 300ml 30% aqueous sodium hydroxide in a 5 litre separating funnel. Run off the lower aqueous phase and reject. Wash the ether phase four times with 300ml distilled water. Finally, distil the ether from 20g solid sodium hydroxide into an amber glass bottle.

Sodium sulphate, anhydrous

Apparatus

Liquid-liquid extractor, upward displacement type, 1 litre capacity, comprising

distributor, extractor tube, boiling flask and condenser, Quickfit and Quartz
Catalogue No. IL RDLU. Round-bottomed, 3-necked, 1 litre flask, with separatory
funnel and connected to horizontally mounted Liebig condenser.

Procedure

To the contents of the extractor containing 800 to 900ml water add 100g solid
sodium chloride. Stir with a glass rod to dissolve the salt as completely as
possible. Charge the extractor with ether and extract for a total period of fifteen
hours. To the flask containing the ether extract, add 3g powdered anhydrous
sodium sulphate powder, and shake to dry the solvent phase. Filter this solution,
in portions, through several layers of Whatman No. 3 filter paper into a 100ml
beaker standing in a warm water bath. Wash the interior of the flask containing
the sodium sulphate with several 25ml portions of fresh ether and transfer these
via the filter paper to the 100ml beaker, ensuring that the whole surface of the
filter paper is washed with ether. Immerse the beaker in a water bath until the
volume of ether is reduced to approximately 10ml. Ensure that no droplets of
water or undissolved organic matter remain in the ether at this stage. Carefully
transfer this solution to a 25ml volumetric flask. Wash the whole interior of
the beaker with several portions of fresh ether and transfer these to the
volumetric flask to make the volume up to 25ml (at 25°C). As soon as possible
transfer to three 25ml beakers, respectively, 6ml and two 8ml portions of the ether
extract by means of a dry 10ml graduated pipette. Apply a nitrogen line to remove
ether completely from the beakers. Use the two beakers containing 8ml of ether
extract for a duplicate determination of sulphur by the Schoniger method described
in Method A. Use the beaker containing 6ml of ether extract for the determination
of dilauryl thiodipropionate by the infra-red spectroscopic method described in
Method B. If there is any delay in continuing the analysis, cover the beakers
with aluminium foil.

Determination of dilauryl thiodipropionate

Method A : Oxygen flask combustion

Reagents

Oxygen cylinder

Sodium hydroxide N/100 - aqueous. Prepare daily by dilution of a standard N/10
stock solution. Ensure that the N/100 sodium hydroxide solution is protected from
contact with atmospheric carbon dioxide as much as possible.

Tashiro mixed indicator

Dissolve 0.125g methyl red in 100ml absolute alcohol. Dissolve 0.083g methylene
blue (B.P. grade) in 100ml absolute alcohol. Use equal volumes of each indicator
for each titration.

Hydrogen peroxide - 100 volume. Microanalytical reagent grade quality, available
from British Drug Houses Ltd., Poole, Dorset.

Percolated water prepared by percolating distilled water through a mixed resin bed
containing Amberlite IR 120H and Amberlite IRA 400 (OH). This water must be
boiled immediately before use and should be used throughout during the Schoniger
combustion stage of the analysis.

Apparatus

Schoniger flasks - 500ml with B24 neck. Platinum wire supports 4 inches long and
fused into B24 stoppers. The free end of the platinum wire is either shaped into
an acute S bend or fitted with a 1 inch square of platinum gauze. Absorbent
ash-free filter paper cut into 1 inch squares.

Graduated burettes - 5ml (Grade A - volumetric glassware)..

To obtain reproducible results by the Schoniger technique it is first advisable
to carry out some combustions of a pure sample of dilauryl thiodipropionate in order
to acquire the necessary experimental skill.

Pipette 1ml of freshly prepared 1% solution of dilauryl thiodipropionate (i.e. 0.01g)
into a 100ml beaker, apply this solution to the paper and carry out the combustion
as described below. Reproducible analysis by this procedure is easily obtained.

Add to a 500ml Schoniger combustion flask 1ml of 100 volume hydrogen peroxide and
10ml of recently boiled-out distilled water. Add 0.1ml each of methyl red and of
methylene blue indicators. Titrate the solution with N/100 sodium hydroxide
solution until it becomes a clear green colour. Fill the flask with pure oxygen
and close immediately with a B24 stopper. To the beaker containing dilauryl
thiodipropionate add 1 to 2ml of ether. Into this solution dip a 1 inch square of
filter paper held by a pair of tweezers. Allow the paper to soak up all the
ether solution. Gently air blowing will evaporate ether from the paper once it
has become saturated. Rinse down the beaker walls with 1 to 2ml of fresh ether
and similarly apply this solution by means of a small glass dropping pipette to
the filter paper. Wash the beaker again with 1 to 2ml ether, and apply the solution
to the filter paper. Allow the filter paper to dry, and fold twice by means of
two pairs of tweezers. Insert the paper between the platinum gauze attached to
the stopper of the Schoniger flask. Into a fold of the paper insert a 2 inch x
1/8 inch strip of filter paper to serve as a wick.

Light the top of the wick and quickly insert into the oxygen-filled combustion
flask. Invert the flask during the combustion (during combustion the operator
should be screened from the flask). Set the flask aside until the mist has
cleared (ten to fifteen minutes). Shake the flask occasionally during this
period. Open the combustion flask and wash down the stopper, wire and neck with
recently boiled-out water. Boil the solution for one minute. Quickly connect a
Carbosorb-filled B24 trap into the mouth of the flask and cool rapidly. Titrate
immediately with N/100 sodium hydroxide to the clear green end-point. Carry out
duplicate blank combustions exactly as described above, except that no sample is
placed on the filter paper. Calculate the dilauryl thiodipropionate content of
the original extraction liquid as described below. Calibrate the procedure as
described below.

Calculate the dilauryl thiodipropionate content of the extraction liquid as
follows:

$$\text{dilauryl thiodipropionate (ppm)(w/v) extraction liquid} = \frac{(T_A - T_B) \times f \times 514 \times 10^6}{2000 \times V}$$

Where T_A = Titration (ml) of sodium hydroxide after Schoniger combustion of
sample extract.

T_B = Titration (ml) of sodium hydroxide after Schoniger combustion of
reagent blank.

V = Volume (ml) of original extraction liquid represented by portion of
ether extract taken for Schoniger combustion.

f = Normality of sodium hydroxide solution.

The method is calibrated against synthetic solutions of dilauryl thiodipiopionate
in the various extraction liquids which have been heated for 10 days at 60°C
and then analysed in exactly the same manner as that used in the case of
extraction liquids obtained in extractability tests carried out on plastics.

Weigh out accurately 0.75g pure dilauryl thiodipropionate into a 100ml beaker and
dissolve in warm absolute ethyl alcohol. Transfer to a 100ml volumetric flask
together with beaker washings and make up to the 100ml mark with alcohol and mix
well. Into five 1 litre ground-glass-stoppered extraction tubes, measure 800ml
of distilled water. Into three further sets of five tubes measure 800ml of the
1:1 ethanol:water extractant, 800ml of the 5% sodium carbonate extractant and
800ml of the 5% citric acid extractant. Into each of the four sets of five tubes,
accurately pipette 0.0, 1.5, 3.5, 7.0 and 10.0ml of 0.75% dilauryl thiodipropionate
in ethyl alcohol, stopper and mix well. Leave the tubes at 60°C for 10 days.
In the case of the five 1:1 ethyl alcohol:water extractants remove alcohol by
distillation and transfer the hot alcohol-free distillation residue to the liquid-
liquid extractor as described above. In the case of the five distilled water,
5% sodium carbonate and 5% citric acid extractants, transfer the hot extractants
to the liquid-liquid extractor as described above. Carry out the ether extraction
of the four sets of extractants and split each of the twenty 25ml ether extracts
into separate portions as described below. Use these solutions to calibrate the
Schoniger procedure and the infra-red procedures as described below.

Determine total sulphur (in duplicate) in 8ml/25ml portions of the twenty ether
extracts by the Schoniger procedure as described above. Calculate the weight of
the dilauryl thiodipropionate equivalent to the determined sulphur content.
Prepare a calibration graph for each of the four extraction liquids by plotting
ppm dilauryl thiodipropionate added to the 800ml of original extraction liquids
(i.e. between 0 and 94 ppm w/v), versus ppm dilauryl thiodipropionate determined
in the 800ml of the original extraction liquid by Schoniger combustion. Use
this calibration graph to determine the sulphur content (i.e. the dilauryl
thiodipropionate content) of the plastic extraction liquids of unknown composition.

Method B : Infra-red spectroscopic method

Reagents

Carbon tetrachloride, spectroscopic grade.

Apparatus

Infra-red spectroscopic - Method B

Infra-red spectrometer, double beam. The Grubb Parsons GS 2A or equivalent
instrument is suitable.

Cells, rock salt 1mm path length.

Volumetric glassware - 10ml flask

Into the beaker containing the ether free extract of the extraction liquid, (see above), pour approximately 5ml spectroscopic grade carbon tetrachloride and swirl to completely dissolve the solid. Transfer this solution quantitatively to a dry 10ml volumetric flask. Wash the walls of the beaker with further small portions of carbon tetrachloride, transfer to the volumetric flask to make up the volume to 10ml and shake the flask well. Transfer a portion of the carbon tetrachloride solution to a 1mm path length rock salt cell, and record its infra-red spectrum in the range 5 to 6 microns. Construct a base line to the dilauryl thiodipropionate peak at 5.75 microns by drawing a straight line between the absorption minima at 5.60 and 5.95 microns and measure the distances I_o and I in millimetres as shown in Figure 60. Calculate the dilauryl thiodipropionate content of the original extraction liquid as described below. Calibrate the procedure as described below.

Calculate the absorbance $(A_{5.75})$ of the 5.75 micron dilauryl thiodipropionate peak as follows:

$$A_{5.75} = Log_{10} \frac{I_o}{I} \quad \cdots \cdots \cdots \quad \text{(see Figure 60)}$$

The dilauryl thiodipropionate content of the original 800ml of extraction liquid in ppm w/v is then obtained by reference to the calibration graph of the absorbance of the 5.75 micron peak vs ppm dilauryl thiodipropionate in 800ml extraction liquid, prepared as described below.

Calibration of the infra-red procedure

Use 6ml/25ml portions of the twenty ether extracts for calibration on the infra-red procedure. Make each of the extracts (ether removed) up to 10ml with spectroscopic grade carbon tetrachloride, and measure the absorbance (in a 1mm path length rock salt cell) of the carbonyl peak occurring at 5.75 microns, as described above. Prepare a calibration graph for each of the four extraction liquids by plotting determined absorbance (A) versus ppm dilauryl thiodipropionate added to 800ml of original extraction liquid (i.e. between 0 and 94 ppm w/v). Use this calibration graph to determine the dilauryl thiodipropionate content of plastic extraction liquids of unknown composition.

Using the above procedures extractability tests have been carried out using the distilled water and the 50% ethyl alcohol:water extractants on 0.001 inch thick polypropylene film containing 0.25% w/w dilauryl thiodipropionate. In these tests the film (31 to 32g) was contacted with 700ml of each extractant for 10 days at 60°C. Each extraction experiment was carried out in duplicate. At the end of the extraction test, dilauryl thiodipropionate was determined in the extractants by the oxygen combustion and the infra-red procedures. The results (Table 36) show that duplicate extraction tests carried out by either method and under identical conditions, gave results which differed by factors of up to ten.

The differences obtained in duplicate extractability tests (Table 36) can be ascribed to a fault in the technique used. In these experiments, the extraction liquid was decanted from the tube after the 10 day heating period, leaving the film in the tube. The tube and its contents was then washed several times with hot water and then diethyl ether to ensure quantitative recovery of dilauryl thiodipropionate. However, separate experiments showed that cold ether can extract considerable quantities of dilauryl thiodipropionate from thin films of polypropylene after a few minutes contact, and it was this which was responsible for the variable extraction test results reported in Table 36. The cold ether polymer washing stage was therefore omitted in the further experiments described below.

TABLE 36

Extractability of dilauryl thiodipropionate from polypropylene

Duplicate extraction tests

Extractant	g dilauryl thiodipropionate extracted/100ml film*		
	by oxygen combustion method		by infra-red method
Distilled water	0.01,	0.01	
Extraction 1	<0.01,	<0.01	<0.01
Extraction 2	0.02,	0.03	0.03
50% ethyl alcohol:water			
Extraction 1	<0.01,	<0.01	0.01
Extraction 2	0.07	0.07	0.07

* calculated according to the method prescribed by the British Plastics Federation[1] for plastic samples less than 0.020 inch thick.

In addition to the factor just discussed, it is believed that the poor agreement obtained in duplicate extraction tests on polypropylene might also be connected with conditions under which the polymer extraction test is carried out. Thus, in the conditions used in the tests (30g film contacted with 700ml extractant as prescribed by the B.P.F.), very poor contact must exist between the large area of film used and the extractant. The film is virtually crushed tightly under extraction liquid in order to bring it beneath the liquid level. This poor contact might cause poor reproducibility in replicate extraction tests.

To examine this point Table 37 shows the results obtained when various volumes of the polypropylene film between 6cm^3 and 34cm^3 were contacted with 700ml of the distilled water extractant which were then left for 10 days at 60°C and shaken periodically. The dilauryl thiodipropionate content of each extraction liquid was then determined by the oxygen combustion method. The results (Table 37) show that within the detection limits of the method, decreasing the ratio volume of film: volume of extractant from 30:700 to 6:700 does not influence the recovery of dilauryl thiodipropionate obtained.

In a further experiment, the polypropylene film (4.4g, 5ml) was wrapped around a stainless steel frame (Figure 61) in such a way that none of the film was in contact. The frame was then immersed in a tank containing 3 litres of distilled water and left for 10 days at 60°C. The water was then concentrated to 500ml by distillation, saturated with sodium chloride and extracted with diethyl ether in a liquid-liquid extractor (the water concentration step was necessary to reduce the volume of the extractant so that it could be conveniently ether-extracted, thereby preserving the sensitivity of the analytical procedure for determining dilauryl thiodipropionate). The dilauryl thiodipropionate content indicated that even under

TABLE 37

Influence of extraction conditions on extractability of
dilauryl thiodipropionate from polypropylene into
the distilled water extractant

Volume (ml) of polymer contacted with 700ml distilled water extractant	g dilauryl thiodipropionate extracted per 100ml polypropylene film
34	< 0.01
34	< 0.01
34	< 0.01
23	< 0.03, 0.04
24	< 0.01
12	< 0.01
12	< 0.01
6	< 0.01
Wire frame method	
5	< 0.01

these very favourable extraction conditions no further extraction of dilauryl thiodipropionate had occurred from the polypropylene film compared with the results obtained in the other experiments referred to in Table 37.

In the Second Toxicity Report[1], the B.P.F. publish an equation for Toxicity Quotient (Q) relating the extractability (E) of an additive from a polymer and the Toxicity Factor (T) of the neat additive, (derived from animal feeding trials)

$$Q = \frac{E \times 1000}{T}$$

Where E = g additive extracted per 100ml polymer volume (for plastic specimens less than 0.020 inch thick).

T = toxicity quotient = 1000 for dilauryl thiodipropionate.

Thus, in the case of dilauryl thiodipropionate

Q = E g additive extracted per 100ml polymer.

The B.P.F. state that for a polymer formulation to be acceptable from the toxicity point of view the sum of the values of Q for the various extractable polymer components shall not exceed 10.

In Table 38 are compared Toxicity Quotients for the extractability of dilauryl thiodipropionate from polypropylene into distilled water, obtained by the oxygen combustion method of analysis and by the thin-layer chromatographic method. Toxicity Quotients determined using the oxygen combustion method and the thin-layer chromatographic method are shown to be of a similar order of magnitude and are considerably below the limit of Q=10. This agreement is very satisfactory considering that these values were determined using completely different analytical procedures.

TABLE 38

B.P.F. Toxicity Quotient of 0.25% dilauryl thiodipropionate in
polypropylene formulations

Extractant:distilled water

Volume of polypropylene film, ml	Volume of distilled water extractant, ml	Ratio volume polymer: volume extractant	Extractability = E g additive extracted per 100ml polymer = Q (Toxicity Quotient)
Oxygen combustion method*			
1.4 (Wire frame method)	200	1:14	<0.01
1.8	200	1:11	<0.01
3.4	200	1:6	<0.01
Thin-layer chromatographic method			
2.1	200	1:10	0.01
2.2	200	1:10	0.01

* Calculated from results in Table 37.

The polypropylene used in these determinations contained 0.25% w/w dilauryl thiodipropionate, i.e. approximately 0.23% w/v. This may be compared with the maximum extractability figure obtained for dilauryl thiodipropionate from this film, namely 0.01g dilauryl thiodipropionate extracted for 100ml film, i.e. 0.01% w/v. It is concluded that a maximum of only 5% of the original additive content of film was extracted into the distilled water extractant during 10 days at 60°C. Dilauryl thiodipropionate does not therefore tend to migrate to any appreciable extent from polypropylene into this extraction liquid. The results in Table 36 show that the migration of the additive into the 50% ethyl alcohol:water extractant is of a similar low order of magnitude to its migration into distilled water.

Chapter 8

Determination of Antioxidants in Foods

For the sake of completeness, this section discusses the determination of various types of antioxidants deliberately added to foods as preservatives. The published work does not mention plastics. No doubt, however, the analyst will find that some of these methods can easily be adapted to the determination in foods of antioxidants that had migrated from plastics in migration tests.

Both butylated hydroxy anisole and butylated hydroxy toluene (2,6,di-tert-butyl-p-cresol) have been used as antioxidants to preserve foods. Phillips[123] described a liquid-liquid extraction of butylated hydroxy toluene and butylated hydroxy anisole from vegetable oils. He studied the partition of butylated hydroxy toluene and butylated hydroxy anisole between heptane and several common polar solvents, and the distribution of ground-nut, maize, soya-bean, and the cotton-seed oils and their influence on antioxidant partition and recommends the following procedure for determining these substances in vegetable oils. Dissolve the sample (4g) in heptane (20ml) and extract with dimethyl sulphoxide (4 × 25ml). Combine the extracts, add water (100ml) and saturated sodium chloride solution (100ml) and extract the mixture with light petroleum (2 × 75ml). Filter the combined extracts and concentrate the filtrate by evaporation. Examine the residue by thin-layer chromatography on silica gel by development with hexane and spraying with Folin-Ciocalteu reagent, or by high-speed liquid chromatography on a 1-metre column of Corasil II, by development with heptane. The latter technique gives 97% recovery of 0.01 to 0.02% of butylated hydroxy toluene in ground-nut oil, and 90±10% recovery at the 0.005% level.

Hartman and Rose[124] described a rapid gas chromatographic method for the determination of butylated hydroxy anisole and butylated hydroxy toluene in vegetable oils. To 2.5g of oil add 150µg of methyl undecanoate (as internal standard) in 5ml of carbon disulphide, and dilute to 25ml with carbon disulphide. Submit a 3 to 7µl aliquot to gas chromatography on an aluminium column (6ft×4.5mm) or a glass column (6ft×4mm) containing 10% of DC200 on gas chrom Q (80 to 100 mesh), operated at 160°C with helium (50ml per min) as carrier gas and flame ionisation detection, and measure the peak areas. To prevent contamination of the columns with non-volatile matter, the aluminium column is fitted with a stainless-steel sleeve containing a 0.25in plug of siliconised glass wool, and the first 4in of the glass column is packed with siliconised glass wool; the glass wool is replaced at the end of each day's analyses. Recoveries of 97 to 104% are obtained for concentrations of 20 to 100ppm of both butylated hydroxy toluene and butylated anisole.

Lemieszek-Chodorowska and Snycerski[125] have described a procedure based on thin-layer chromatography for the detection of phenolic antioxidants in edible fats and in oils. In this procedure the sample (10g) is dissolved in light petroleum (25ml) at 50% and extracted with 72% ethanol (3 × 5ml), shaking for 5min each time. Evaporate the combined ethanolic extracts at 20°C dissolve the residue in 96% ethanol (0.5ml) and apply this solution to 0.25mm silical gel layers that have been activated at 105° for 1 hour. Develop the chromatograms with chloroform, anhydrous acetic acid (17:3) for separating propyl gallate, octyl gallate, dodecyl gallate and nordihydroguaiaretic acid, or with chloroform for separating butylated hydroxy anisole and 2,6-di-t-butyl-p-cresol. Dry the chromatogram and reveal the spots by spraying it with 1% silver nitrate solution in 25% aqueous ammonia and heating at 70°C to 80°C for 20 min. This method permits the detection of as little as 0.5µg of propyl gallate, 1µg of octyl and dodecyl gallates and nordihydrog-uaiaretic acid and butylated hydroxy anisole and 3µg 2,6-di-tert-butyl-p-cresol.

2,6-di-tert-butyl-p-cresol, butylated hydroxy anisole, propyl gallate and tocophenol can be determined in fats extracted from mayonnaise, biscuits or margarine by thin-layer chromatography on layers of (0.5mm) of silica gel activated at 105°C for 1 hour. Development is with chloroform, spots are located by spraying the air-dried chromatogram with 10% ethanolic molybdophosphoric acid, and the coloured zones are compared with those of antioxidant standards (Vicente et al[126], Schwein and Conroy[127]).

Thin-layer chromatography on polyamide-kieselguhr has been used to separate fat antioxidants (Chiang and Tseng[128]). The separation of propyl, isoamyl, lauryl, hexadecyl and stearyl gallates, t-butyl-4-methoxyphenol, 2,6-di-t-butyl-p-cresol and ethyl protocatechuate is described by these workers. Using a thin layer of nylon 6-Kieselguhr G (2:1), they apply the antioxidants as a 0.5% solution in ethanol, and develop with one of the following solvents – isoamyl alcohol for 9 hours; isoamyl acetate-acetone (5:1) for 2 hours; isoamyl acetate-xylene-ethanol (20:1:1) for 2.5 hours; acetone-water (5:3) for 2.5 hours; or dioxan water-ethanol (10:7:5) for 3 hours. The spots are revealed by spraying the chromatogram with 0.07% ethanolic Rhodamine B (C.I. Basic Violet 10) and examination in ultra-violet radiation, and by exposure to iodine vapour. Lehman and Moran[129] used a micro-column of polyamide powder in the analysis of antioxidants in fats. The antioxidants were extracted from a light petroleum solution of the fat by acetonitrile, or were adsorbed from the fat on to Celite (light petroleum as solvent) and extracted with methanol. They were then separated into two groups on a micro-column of polyamide powder, on which gallate esters, dihydrocaffeic acid and nordihydroguaiaretic acid were adsorbed from 70% methanol medium. The column was washed with water and 70% methanol, and ascorbyl acetate, t-butyl-4-methoxyphenol, 2,6-di-t-butyl-p-cresol, guaiacol and tocopherols in the percolate and washings were separated by thin-layer chromatography and identified. The adsorbed antioxidants were then eluted with methanolic sodium hydroxide and, after acidifying the eluate were separated by thin-layer chromatography and identified.

To determine antioxidants in food oils Vigneron and Spicht[130] extracted an hexane solution of the oil with 1% ammonium acetate, 32% aqueous acetonitrile and 48% aqueous acetonitrile to respectively isolate propyl, octyl and dodecyl gallates. As traces of t-butyl-4-methoxyphenol are also extracted by the last solvent, a hexane solution of another portion of the sample was extracted with 30% water (to remove the gallates) and washed with aqueous ammonia, then the tert-butyl-4-methoxyphenol is extracted with 72% aqueous ethanol; 2,6-di-t-butyl-p-cresol remains in the hexane solution.

Pino et al[131] carried out a comparative study of chromatographic and colorimetric methods for the identification of phenolic antioxidants in edible fats. They claim that the best solvent for extracting the antioxidants from the oil is aceto-nitrile saturated with light petroleum (bp 40° to 60°C). The best separation is

obtained on layers of polyamide powder with light petroleum-benzene-acetic acid-
dimethylformamide (40:40:20:1) as solvent, but acceptable results are obtained on
silica gel layers with a similar solvent without the dimethylformamide. For
locating the spots, 0.5% ethanolic 2,5-dichloro-p-benzoquinonechlorimine is
suitable. The only permitted phenolic antioxidant not identifiable in this way
is butylated hydroxy toluene, which may be separated by steam-distillation and detected
colorimetrically with o-dianisidine-nitrous acid. In this distillate, butylated
hydroxy anisole may be confirmed by a colour test with 3,5-dichloro-p-benzoquinone-
chlorimine.

McBride and Evans[132] developed a rapid voltametric method for the estimation of
antioxidants and tocopherols in oils and fats. The sample solutions were prepared
by dissolving the oil or lard sample in an appropriate solvent, e.g. in most
instances 0.12M-sulphuric acid in ethanol-benzene (2:1). The solutions were analysed
with use of a linearly varying potential and a stationary, planar vitreous-carbon
electrode, with a S.C.E. and a platinum-wire counter-electrode. Separate peaks were
obtained for α-, γ- and δ- tocopherol: the peak for the β-isomer, was superimposed
on that for the γ-tocopherol. Butylated hydroxy anisole (>10ppm) can be determined
in vegetable oil under the same conditions, provided that δ-tocopherol is absent.
Kohler et al[133] described a polarographic method for the determination of 4-4'
thiobis(6-tert-butyl-m-cresol) in food. The antioxidant is first nitrated,
p r eferably with fuming nitric acid-conc sulphuric acid (1:1) at 20 for 1 hour.
The polarography is carried out on the resulting solution after dilution and
addition of urea and sodium acetate buffer solution. The $E_\frac{1}{2}$ for the nitrated
compound is -0.54V vs. the mercury pool. The limit of the determination is 0.02μg
per ml with a cathode-ray polarograph or 1μg per ml with a conventional d.c.
polarograph.

Takahashi[134][135] used gas liquid chromatography to determine butylated hydroxy
anisole and butylated hydroxy toluene (2,6-di-tert-butyl-p-cresol) in breakfast
cereals. He claims quantitative recoveries of from 20 to 30 ppm of the antioxidants
added to cereals. To determine antioxidants and preservatives in soya sauce and
other foods Takemura[136] converted these compounds to trimethylsilyl derivatives
and analysed the product by gas chromatography. The sample was shaken with the
silation reagent (1ml) for 30seconds, then set aside for 5 minutes and 2μl of
the solution was analysed by gas chromatography on, e.g. 20% of SE-31 silicone on
Celite 545 at 200°C with helium (22ml per min) as carrier gas and hexane as
internal standard. The method was applied to 15 perservatives and 7 antioxidants;
well-separated peaks are obtained for 4-hydroxybenzoate esters, phenol, xylenol
derivatives and salicylic acid. The calibration graphs for methyl,ethyl, propyl
and butyl 4-hydroxybenzoates are rectilinear for the range 0.5 to 4mg. The method
was used to determine 4-hydroxybenzoates in soya sauce.

Halat[137]has reviewed methods of separating, detecting and determining six
commercially used antioxidants in foods at concentrations down to 0.01%.
Lee[138][138] has described procedures for the detection of additives in foodstuffs
utilizing thin-layer chromatography. Ethyl protocatechuate, propyl isoamyl, lauryl
cetyl and stearyl gallates, t-butyl methoxyphenol and 2,6-di-t-butyl-p-cresol are
separated on layers (0.25mm) of polyamide-silica gel (8:15) by development with a
1:4 mixture of anhydrous acetic acid with chloroform, benzene or carbon tetrachloride.
The dried chromatograms are sprayed with ammoniacal to silver nitrate solution to
locate the antioxidants as light-brown to black spots. The limits of detection
range from 9.05 to 2μg. The method was applied to butter and lard.

Various other workers have studied methods for the determination of antioxidants
in fats and foods. These include Roos[140], Biefer and Hadorn[141], Gander[142][143]
Brown and Blaxter[144][145]ter Heide[146], Zipp[147]and Stahl[148]. Biefer and Hadorn[141]
used paper chromatography to separate tocopherols from fats and Gander[142][143]
applied this technique, somewhat unsuccessfully, to the determination of antioxidants
in fats. Brown and Blaxter[144][145] and ter Heide[146] studied the application of

different solvent extraction systems to the separation of antioxidants from fats.
Stahl[148] was one of the first to apply thin-layer chromatography to the separation
of antioxidants from fats.

Seher[149 150] carried out an extensive study of the applicability of thin-layer
chromatography on 250-300μ thick layers of silica gel to the identification of
naturally occuring and added synthetic antioxidants in fats (Table 39). Colour
reactions for the location of separated compounds on the thin-layer plate are
included in this Table. Phosphomolybdic acid proved to be the most sensitive
chromogenic reagent.

To identify the separated compounds Seher[149 150] sprayed the air dried plates
with a 20% solution of phosphomolybdic acid in ethanol or ethylene glycol momomethyl
ether (methyl "Cellosolve") until they become a uniform yellow. The first antioxidants appear as blue spots within the first one or two minutes. The plate is
then treated with ammonia vapour which causes the substrate to turn pure white
while the substances stand out very clearly as dark blue, in some cases violet
or greenish tinged spots.

Compounds with a poor reducing action also turn molybednum blue within ten minutes,
if the plate is heated in the drying cupboard to 120°C.

Compounds which can be identified by this process are listed in Table 39. The
lower identification limit in the complete thin-layer chromatogram was ascertained
as about 1μg per spot (Figure 62).

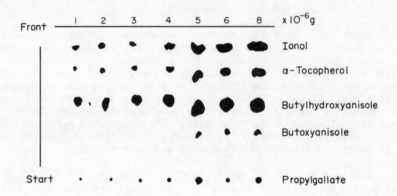

FIG.62 Thin-layer chromatographic separation of antioxidants using phosphomolybdic
        acid as chromogenic reagent and chloroform as eluant.

Seher[150] found that reacting antioxidants with 2,6 dichloroquinone chlorimide was
unspecific. Even though only a few of the compounds tested turned blue, the
formation of coloured products in the thin-layer chromatogram could be proved with
all antioxidants tested. The colours obtained are listed in Table 39. The air-dried
chromatogram is sprayed uniformly with a 1% solution of 2,6-dichloroquinone
chlorimide in ethanol. When left in a neutral atmosphere, coloured spots become
visible with 15 minutes. When subsequently resprayed with a 20% borax solution in
40% ethanol some of the products show the characteristic colour changes given in

TABLE 39

List of Antioxidants tested and their behaviour towards various Identification Reagents(Seher151 152)

Plates: silica gel, dried at 120°C, eluted with chloroform then dried at 120°C for 10 mins and stored in desiccator

No	Compound	Phospho-molybdic acid	2,6 dichloroquinone chlorimide		diazotised sulphanilic acid
			neutral	borate buffer	
1	α-tocopherol	+	yellowish-brown	yellowish-brown	—
2	α-tocopherol-acetate	—	pink	(pink)	—
3	2,2,5,7,8-pentamethyl-6-hydroxy-chromane	+	brownish-yellow	yellowish-brown	—
4	Propyl-gallate	+	brown	greyish-brown	brownish-red
5	Octyl-gallate	+	brown	greyish-brown	brownish-red
6	Dodecyl-gallate	+	brown	greyish-brown	brownish-red
7	2-tert.butyl-4-hydroxyanisole	+	rust-brown	violet	pink
8	3-tert.butyl-4-hydroxyanisole	+	rust-brown	violet	pink
9	2,5-di-tert.butyl-4-hydroxyanisole	+	purple	violet	—
10	3-tert.butyl-4-hydroxytoluene	+	orange	orange	yellow
11	3,5-di-tert.butyl-4-hydroxytoluene	+	yellow	(light yellow)	yellow
12	Nordihydroguaiaretic acid	+	violet	brownish-violet	carmine-red
13	Guaiacum	+	olive-green	olive-green	dark brown
14	Ascorbyl palmitate	+	red	pale-violet	—
15	Hydroquinone monomethylether	+	reddish-violet	blue-violet	orange
16	4-tert.butoxy-anisole	+	reddish-violet	blue-violet	—
17	Monoglyceride-citrate	(+)*	pink	pale violet	—
18	N.lauroyl-p-phenetidine	—	pale pink	pale pink	yellowish-brown
19	N-stearoyl-p-phenetidine	+	pale pink	pale pink	yellowish-brown
20	N,N'-diphenyl-p-phenylenediamine	+	greyish-brown	greyish-brown	canary-yellow
21	Tetraethyl-thiuramdisulphide	+	rust-brown	brown	—
22	β-β'-thio-di-propionic acid	+	pale brown	orange	—
23	4-n-butylmercapto-butanone-(2)	+	canary yellow	pale brown	—
24	2,4,6-tri-tert.butyl-phenol	+	orange	purple	—

*Reaction only takes place on heating.

Table 39 which can be used as an additional aid to identification.

Treatment with ammonia vapour provides no great advantage as it causes the substrate to take on a darker colour.

As these methods can only be used for reducing compounds, i.e. unchanged antioxidants Seher[150] attempted to find another reaction which would make it possible to identify conversion products of the antioxidants which form during storage of the fat. Aromatic compounds can be coupled with diazotized sulphanilic acid to form dyes. The shades are given in Table 39.

Seher[150] studied both one dimentional and two dimentional solvent elution of the thin-layer plate in an attempt to fully resolve complex mixtures of antioxidants separated from fats. Table 40 shows the eluting agents tested and their properties.

TABLE 40

The Effects and Suitability of Different Eluting Agents

Eluting Agent	Eluting Effect	Suitability for Separation
Hexane		Almost all substances at the starting point
Tetrachloroethylene		
Carbon Tetrachloride		
Toluene		Good spot formation
Benzene		
Methyl "Cellosolve"		All substances in the front
Dioxane		
Methylene chloride		
Ethyl acetate		Unsuitable because too much tail formation
Nitromethane		
Acetone		
Methanol		
i-propanol		

Figure 63 shows the migration of some of the tested antioxidants when eluted with chloroform. It can be seen from this figure that well-defined spots were formed. It can be seen from the chromatogram of the same mixture of substances that it is not possible to separate the individual components satisfactorily with chloroform nor indeed with any of the other eluting agents. Although none of the eluting agents tested can alone achieve satisfactory separation, the migration paths are sufficiently differentiated using various solvents to make it possible to obtain satisfactory separation by a two-dimensional procedure. Optimum success is

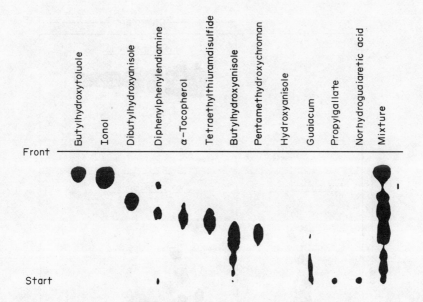

FIG.63 Thin-layer chromatographic separation of antioxidants using chloroform as
        eluant.

obtained by elution with chloroform in one direction and benzene in the second
direction. Figure 64 shows the effect of this method, using the mixture shown in
Fig. 63.

The procedure finally evolved by Seher[151] is described below.

The mixture to be separated was applied at three starting points and then eluted
with chloroform (the horizontal direction in the Figure). After a front 10cm
above the starting point had been reached, the plate was dried in the air for 10
mins, and elution was then continued with benzene after the plate had been turned
through 90° (the vertical direction in the Figure). Here too, elution was ended
after a front 10cm above the starting point had been reached. The plate was dried
in the air for 5 mins and then sprayed with phosphomolybdic acid in the described
manner.

By applying three samples of the mixture at three different spots on the plate
simultaneously, separation is achieved by each eluting agent both in one direction
alone and by the two-dimensional method (Figure 64). It is possible to distinguish
between the following compounds:

Ionol; dibutylhydroxy anisole; diphenyl-p-phenylenediamine; α-tocopherol- tetraethyl-
thiuram disulphide; pentamethyl-hydroxychromane; butylated hydroxyanisole;
monoglyceride citrate; butoxyanisole; guaiacum; gallates (+ nordihydroguaiaretic
acid + ascorbyl palmitate).

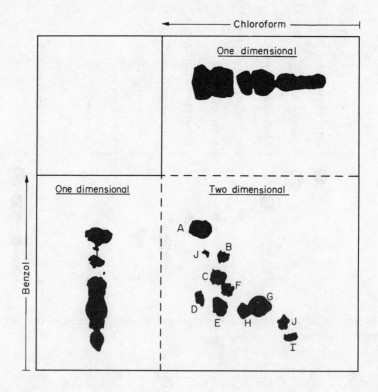

FIG.64   Separation of antioxidants by two-dimentional thin-layer chromatography.

    A = Ionol
    B = Dibutyl hydroxy anisole
    C = Diphenyl-p-benylene diamine (J impurity in C)
    D = Monoglyceride citrate
    E = Tetraethylthiuram sulphide
    F = α-Tocopherol
    G = Butylated hydroxy anisole
    H = Pentamethyl hydroxy chromane
    I = Guaiacum
    J = Butoxy hydroxy anisole

Chapter 9

Legislative Aspects of the Use of Additives
in Foodgrade Plastics

In this Chapter is reviewed the legislation pertaining to the use of additives in foodgrade plastics in various countries. The legislation is reviewed and also the method of its implementation and the procedure that must be followed by anyone who wishes to seek approval for the use of any polymer or additive in applications involving contact with foodstuffs.

The situation in the following countries is reviewed in some detail; United Kingdom, British Commonwealth, United States of America, France Italy, West Germany, Sweden, Switzerland, Belgium, Holland, Norway, Denmark and Spain. The situation in the following countries is reviewed more briefly; Austria and East Europe, Canada, Australia, New Zealand, South Africa, India, Japan and Latin America.

The harmonisation of legislation in the EEC is proceeding steadily. The Council of Europe has tended to concentrate its efforts on intrinsic toxicity of additives. The EEC has been studying the legal aspects of the harmonisation of legislation since 1963 and has also been studying migration of additives. Draft EEC regulations are now actively under discussion, although it will probably take several years to finalize the documents and promulgate them within the nine countries concerned.

United Kingdom

In the United Kingdom, packaging and plastics in contact with food, from the health point of view, are covered by Common Law. The relevant statute law is the Food and Drugs Act 1955. This Act gives wide powers to the relevant ministers to issue regulations covering food quality in all its aspects including packaging. Although, no legislation or regulations exist which refer specifically to packaging or plastics it is, nevertheless, possible to bring packaging into the orbit of the 1955 Act by regarding packaging or food contact as a source of adventitious food additive, i.e. if a plastics transmitted a foreign substance to a food thereby contaminating, adulterating or tainting it or making it unsafe for consumption, the food would be deemed to infringe the Act and the plastics contacting it held to blame. In addition, certain sections of the Act directly cover food packaging; (Sections 1(1), 1(3) and 2, 1955 Act). These sections refer specifically to

food being made injurious to health, and food which is not of the nature, substance
or quality demanded by the purchaser and this would include quality aspects such as
tainting and off-flavours.

Under British law it is only retailers or distributors of food that can be
prosecuted. The plastics producer is safe from prosecution unless he packaged
the food himself, or gave false assurances that the food container was suitable for
use with food when he had reason to believe that this was not so.

Details of the 1955 Act are filled in by the issue of regulations, several of which
have been issued. Thus, the Antioxidant in Food Regulations 1955, the colouring
matter in Food Regulations 1957, the Mineral Oil in Food Regulations 1949 and the
amended Preservatives in Food Regulations 1925. All these regulations provide a
positive list of approved additives or food components with maximum concentrations,
all others being banned. Thus, if, for example a banned antioxidant migrated from
a plastics container into a food in significant quantities there would be an
infringement of the regulations. To date, there has not been a prosecution
connected with plastics under these regulations.

In the implementation of the 1955 Act, ministers are advised by two committees,
the Food Standards Committee, which is concerned with composition and descriptive
matter (labelling) and the Food Additives and Contaminants Committee (FACC).
Implementation of the statute law is also carried out by local authorities with the
Public Analyst as a key figure exactly as occurs in the case of common law.

As far as plastics in contact with food is concerned, statute law reinforces
common law. It is necessary for a plastics merchant to satisfy himself that no
health hazard will arise from the use of his product and that he can prove in court
that he has carried out trials to prove this, or he has used the best available
advice or both.

In the United Kingdom, if such trials are necessary, it is common for plastics
merchants to arrange for such trials to be carried out jointly on behalf of the
whole industry by the British Plastics Federation(BPF) who operate a scheme for
conducting such joint trials. The results of the BPF are published in "Plastics
for Food Contact Applications - A Code of Practice for Safety in Use". Toxicity
assessments of additives are carried out by the British Industrial Biological
Research Association (BIBRA). Alternative sources of best available advice are
other published data by recognised authorities and non-U.K. statutory approvals
such as are allowed by legislation in the U.S.A., West Germany and Holland.

To summarise, therefore, a merchant of food contact plastics in the U.K. should
conform to his customers requirements and conform to the BPF/BIBRA Code of Practice
or carry out his own trials to satisfy himself of safety, or adhere strictly to
U.S.A., West German or Dutch legislation.

British Commonwealth

In general, the Commonwealth adopts the U.K. legislation with perhaps special
regulations to cover local situations. However, some members of the Commonwealth
have independent legislative systems which may be different from the U.K. one.

United States of America

As the United States legislation has been adopted outright or in a modified form

by many other countries this legislation is discussed below in some detail.   In
the United States food law is strongly inclined to statute law.   Although, each
State can legislate separately, in practice the federal law usually prevails which
has considerable advantages in inter-state commerce.   Many states have their own
laws which are identical to the federal law.

The principal United States law is the Food, Drug and Cosmetic Act (1938).   This
law is designed to "provide food safe and wholesome to the people, honestly
labelled and properly packaged".   Packaging in relation to health was brought into
the Act, which is current, by an amendment issued in 1955 (Food Additive Amendment).

This Amendment states:

1.   The burden of proof of safety "to the health of man or animal" of a food additive
     is placed on the person causing the addition.

2.   The Secretary of the Health, Education and Welfare Department (HEW), acting
     on the advice of the Food and Drugs Administration (FDA) is authorised to
     "prescribe the conditions under which an additive may be safely used".

3.   The Delaney Amendment overrides the Health, Education and Welfare Department
     and absolutely prohibits use at any concentration of an additive which induces
     cancer in man or animal.

4.   Regarding definition of a food additive; these are any substances the intended
     use of which results in may be reasonably be expected to result, directly or
     indirectly, in its becoming a component or otherwise affecting the characteristics
     of any food including any substance intended for use in producing, manufacturing,
     packaging, processing, preparing, treating, transporting or holding food ......

5.   A substance may be exempted from such control if it is:

     a) 'generally recognised among experts, qualified by scientific training or
        experience to evaluate its safety, as having been adequately shown,
        through scientific procedures (or in the case of a substance used in food
        prior to January 1st, 1958 through scientific procedures or experience
        based on common use in food), to be safe under the conditions of its intended
        use', or

     b) 'used in accordance with a sanction or approval granted prior to the
        enactment of the Amendment, or under the similar clause in the Poultry
        Products Inspection, or Meat Inspection Acts as amended'.

In the United States, therefore, the use of plastics in contact with food is under
the direct jurisdiction of the Food and Drug Administration who issue detailed
positive lists of permitted plastics and additives.   The whole cost of test and
evaluation is put on the plastics and additive manufacturers.   The Delaney
Amendment has caused great difficulty but has not yet affected plastics.

The positive list of plastics and additives has three categories.   Generally
recognised as safe (some additives approved under this category) prior sanction
(i.e. prior to January 1st, 1958) all others (this includes approval of most
base plastics).

In the packaging of meat and poultry, surveillance of packaging materials is
covered   by the Meat Inspection Act (1907).

The FDA regulations are held in great respect throughout the world.   Other
countries tend to follow them, often in a simplified form.

The 1958 Amendment to the Food, Drug and Cosmetic Act specifies that the following information must be supplied to the FDA by the company wishing to market or manufacture when making an application for approval of a plastic or an additive for use in contact with food:

1. Composition
2. Conditions of use and labelling
3. "All relevant data bearing on the physical or technical effect such additive is intended to produce and quantity of such additive required to produce such effect"
4. Analytical methods.
5. Toxicity data.

The FDA itself in the guidelines indicate that they require information on composition, usage, toxicity and migration.

If a petition to the FDA to use an additive or plastic is approved, this fact is published in the FDA Bulletin, together with information on (1) the types of additives and plastics, (2) the types of food that may be packaged and (3) conditions of use of package.

(1) Types of plastic and additive.

    a) Base plastics,
    b) Individual additives for prescribed uses,
    c) Additives for use in specific packaging materials,
    d) Additives or materials used for a specific technological reason, e.g. lubricants.

(2) Types of food.

    a) Non-acid, aqueous, pH greater than 5 may contain salt or sugar or both.
    b) Acid aqueous, may contain salt or sugar or both and including oil-in-water emulsions low or high fat content.
    c) Aqueous acid or non-acid with free oil or fat, may contain salt, and include oil or water or emulsions of these – low or high fat.
    d) i) Water in oil emulsions, high or low fat,
       ii) Oil in water emulsions, high or low fat,
    e) Low moisture fats and oils,
    f) Beverages,
       i) Up to 8% alcohol,
      ii) Non-alcoholic,
    iii) More than 8% alcohol,
    g) Bakery goods other than those covered by types 1 and 2,
      i) Moist bakery products, surface containing free fat or oil,
      ii) Similar , with no free fat or oil,
    h) Dry solids – surface containing no free fat or oil,
    i) Dry solids – surface containing free fat or oil,

(3) Conditions of use of package,
    a) High temperature heat stabilised,
    b) Boiling water sterilised (e.g. up to 100°C),
    c) Hot filled, or pasteurised, above 150°C,
    d) Hot filled, or pasteurised below 150°C,
    e) Room temperature filled or stored (no thermal treatment in container),
    f) Refrigerated storage (no thermal treatment in container),
    g) Frozen storage (no thermal treatment in container),
    h) Frozen or refrigerated storage. Including ready prepared foods intended to be reheated in container at time of use:
      i) Aqueous or oil-in-water emulsion of high or low fat,
      ii) Aqueous, high or low free oil or fat.

The outcome of such legislation is that rarely is general approval given to the use of particular additives and plastics. The approval is hedged with restrictions which qualify it quoting types of food and conditions of use.

To market in or export to the United States it is essential to conform to FDA regulations and in the case of packaged meat and poultry, United States Department of Agriculture Regulations (USDA). The merchant who intends to use the plastic should seek a written guarantee from the supplier of plastics raw material that it conforms with the regulations for its intended use.

The plastics manufacturer must consider his product from the points of view of basic polymer, additives/adjuvants and migration of anything from the plastic into the packaged commodity.

The base polymer must conform to the FDA or USDA specifications. All additives must similarly conform and any restrictions with regard to foods and conditions of use complied with. In this connection it is usually necessary for the plastics producer to seek a guarantee from the additive manufacturer or supplier that his material (i.e. the neat additive) is of the quality specified in the FDA (or USDA) regulations.

The polymer manufacturer must be satisfied that the additives present in his polymer meet any migration limits specified in the regulations.

France

In France the main decree covering all materials and objects in contact with food came into force in February 1973 and February 1974 (decree No 73-138). Its main relevant provisions are discussed below.

Article 2 (February 1973) provides that materials or objects contacting food must be "inert with regard to foodstuffs". In particular, they "must not cede, in their various conditions of use, any amount of elements susceptible of abnormally modifying the composition of the food, notably in conferring on it a poisonous character, or altering its organoleptic quality". The suitability of materials in this context is to be verified by a method specified in a statutory order issued jointly by the Ministers of Agriculture and Rural Development, Economy and Finance, Public Health, and of Industrial and Scientific Development, following advice from the Conseil Superieur d'Hygiene Publique de France. This Article also states that it is necessary for "the Statutory Order to fix the maximum limit above which the composition of the foodstuff is abnormally modified".

Article 3 (February 1973) provides that materials and objects containing food must be made exclusively from constituents whose presence does not give rise to a health risk. It is intended to set up a positive list of such substances which will specify:

   i) criteria of purity,
  ii) conditions of use,
 iii) the maximum concentration tolerable in the food.

Article 4 (February 1973) prohibits irradiation except under conditions defined in current relevant French regulations.

Article 5 (February 1974) deals with labelling which must specify whether the packaging material is suitable for general use or for a restricted stated range of foods.

Article 6 (February 1975) exempts from Article 5 objects such as cooking utensils
which are obviously intended for food usage.

Article 7 (February 1975) states that it is necessary to indelibly indicate the
fact on plastics which are unsuitable for food packaging or contact.

Article 9 deals with mineral and table water bottles, baby feeding bottles, teats
and dummies.

Articles 14-17 cover the legal details necessary to fit the decree into the basic
law of France.

The principle underlying these regulations is that anything migrating from packaging
into food is a food contaminant; it must, therefore, either be approved as such or
the migration must not constitute a toxic hazard or exhibit tainting. The latter
requirement can be satisfied by either demonstrating zero migration or its inclusion
in a positive list. The basis for inclusion of materials on the positive list is
given in a circular letter of 12 September 1963.

Administration of these statutes is carried out by the Répression des Fraudes
which authority has police powers but does not carry out basic investigations into
additives.

In view of the fact that the latest French laws regarding the use of plastics
additives have only been in existence since February 1973, the full effects of
these laws have not yet been felt by plastics manufacturers, nor will they be for
some time.

Italy

Contemporary legislation in Italy is Article 11 of Law N283, (April 1962) which
deals with all aspects of food safety, and authorises detailed administration by
ministerial decree. The decrees relevant to food packaging were issued in 1963
and replaced by further laws between 1966 and 1973. The current decree is N104
of 20 April 1973, covering all packaging materials.

The decrees mentioned above are issued by Ministers and published in the Gazette
Ufficiale. Decree N104 covers all "materials which are destined to come into
contact with foodstuffs or substances for personal use".

Articles 1 to 9 deal with definitions, scope and application. It provides that
food contacting materials "may only be prepared with the ingredients specified ...
subject to conditions... of use stated". New ingredients must be approved by the
Ministry of Health (Article 4). Article 5 provides for a "global migration" limit
of 50ppm in food simulant for objects larger than 250ml, and 8 mg/dm^2 for smaller
articles. Article 6 places responsibility on the "companies which manufacture
objects" to ensure compliance and states that "each consignment must be accompanied
by a declaration by the manufacturer stating that the objects ... comply with the
standards currently in force". Article 7 indicates that the objects covered by the
decree should be "technically suitable for the field of application for which they
are intended", and that "the company should be provided with a declaration of
conformity issued by the manufacturer ... so that they are always in a position to
help the health authorities identify the supplier or manufacturer of the object".
Article 8 covers labelling and requires that the words "for foodstuffs" is
displayed and any restrictions stated. Article 9 allows only approved plastic
compositions and Article 10 states that they must conform to stipulated tests and
that they "must in no way cede substances considered harmful to health such as

monomers, low molecular weight compounds, intermediates, catalysts, solvents and emulsifying agents". Article 11 states that plastic objects must be checked for "global migration" using specified methods involving contact with simulant liquids for 10 days at 40°C and for 2 hours at 80°C. Article 12 allows "any colouring agents" provided that they "do not migrate into the foodstuff" and are below the following limits for heavy metals and primary amines:

Lead	0.01%
Arsenic	0.005%
Mercury	0.005% in N/10 HCℓ
Cadmium	0.20% in N/10 HCℓ
Selenium	0.01% in N/10 HCℓ
Barium	0.01% in N/10 HCℓ
Free primary amines 0.05%	

Articles 13 and 14, respectively, prohibit use of the scrap of recycle plastics and the use of plastics pipes for drinking and mineral water. The Appendices include full details of analytical methods and a positive list for additives.

Thus, in Italy, conformity with the legislation is mandatory. The following requirements must be met by the plastics merchant:

1. "global migration" limit,

2. conformity with positive list,

3. adequate labelling,

4. general safety in use.

If a merchant wishes to use a non-approved additive or plastics he must first seek approval and wait until this has been officially published before marketing can take place.

West Germany

The relevant law dates from 1936 and covers utensils, which are defined to include packaging and all materials coming into direct contact with foodstuffs or beverages. This law was amended in 1958 (Bundesgesetzblatt 1958, I p.950) to bring in definite association with packaging materials. This forbade foreign materials and defined these as those which do not contain digestible carbohydrates, fats or which contain these in amounts which are not useful in food. Under the 1958 amendment migrants are only permitted if they:

1. present no toxic hazard

2. do not taint the food,

3. are technically unavoidable.

No mandatory specifications are issued in West Germany which are binding legislation but the Federal Health Office (Bundesgesundheitamt) publishes recommendations that are widely accepted. Modifications to legislation are currently under active consideration in West Germany.

The recommendations of the Bundesgesundheitamt are made on the advice of the Kunstoffkommissi on, which is a joint committee of civil servants and industry. This committee makes no recommendations itself but examines data on migration and

toxicity presented to it. All their recommendations are published separately and
in collective volumes (Kunststoffe im Lebensmittelverkehr, Karl Heymans, Verlag).

There is no direct policing. The responsibility for the general administration of
public health rests with the various State Health Authorities. Infringment of the
law requires non-conformity with Bundesgesundheitamt regulations and some
demonstrable hazard such as taint or lack of need of the inclusion of the additive
in the plastic formulation.

Plastic merchants in West Germany would usually only consider deviations from the
Bundesgesundheitamt recommendations if such deviation is unavoidable, or technical
need can be proven or no health hazard can be proved convincingly.

When a new plastic or additive is concerned approval should be sought from the
Kunststoffkommission in Berlin with a view to a recommendation being published.
Information would be required regarding full details of the product, migration
tests with foodstuff simulants and toxiological data. Technoligical need for
plastic or additive and freedom from tainting are also investigated in such
applications.

Sweden

The most recent relevant Act in Sweden was issued in 1971 and it is similar to the
Food and Drugs Act of the United Kingdom. It provides that food deemed injurious
to consumer or which is infected or otherwise unfit for human consumption, may not
be offered for sale. Only approved additives may be used. This law specifically
prohibits foods containing foreign substances exceeding a certain quantity and
covers contaminants such as heavy metals and adventicious additives arising from
food packaging materials.

Switzerland

The basic current legislation is the Federal Food Laws of 1905 which deal with food
quality and standards and provides for packaging materials and food utensils.
It was followed by the decree of 1936 (No. 450, Section 7) covering food contact
materials, and 1957 (No. 65, Section 10) specifically dealing with meat packaging.
These decrees state that only approved materials, including plastics, may be used
in contact with food. To be approved, the food contact material must not introduce
toxic hazard into the food, nor must it taint it.

The decrees mentioned above provide for the creation of positive lists and specifications and such lists have already been issued for foodstuffs themselves and
their additives. In August 1969, a draft positive list was drawn up for plastics.
This list has not yet, however, been issued. In its place a licensing system has
been adopted, whereby health authorities in each canton authorise use in contact
with food of plastics and all necessary investigations are carried out by the
health authority at Berne.

Information required from the plastic manufacturer and end user by these
authorities includes data on composition, migration, toxicity, foreign approvals and
conditions of usage. The authorities rely on this information but do carry out some
migration testing and organoleptic trials.

Permission to use plastics for food contact in Switzerland comes from the Berne
cantonal health authority.

Belgium

The current law (No. 135, 1964) states that is is forbidden to market any foodstuff containing additives not previously authorised by the Ministry of Health or containing an additive above the level permitted. The law clearly distinguishes between intentional additives (e.g. deliberately added food preservatives) and unintentional additives (e.g. substances migrated from plastic packages).

Various decrees have been issued under this frame law. The most relevant to plastics packaging is that issued in October 1972. From the point of view of health safety the most important Section of this decree is Article 4 which states that food contact materials must not "cede constituent elements in a quantity or a fashion such that the material contacted, or food substance, becomes or may become dangerous or harmful to health".

No positive lists have yet been issued in Belgium for packaging materials including plastics.

Detailed implementation of the law is by the Department of Public Health.

Holland

The earlier food laws in Holland were amplified in 1955 (Official Gazette No. 481) by a general order dealing with food packaging. This states that the packaging should not transmit to the food components which might be detrimental to health. Between 1963 and 1973 draft packaging regulations with emphasis on plastics were published for comment including positive lists. None of these has yet been promulgated. In particular, the 1968 law envisages permitted use based on migration data alone but would require an extremely low migration rate of less than 0.05ppm in food.

Policing of the law is by food inspectors assisted by provincial and municipal laboratories. Although the law is not yet mandatory, the draft regulations are accepted in Holland and operate in an equivalent manner to the Code of Practice in the United Kingdom and West Germany. A merchant who wishes to use an additive or a new plastic not currently approved would provide information to prove neglibible migration into foodstuff simulants or provide a 6 day migration test data to show that the migration does not exceed safe limits.

Norway

A committee has been set up to consider the implications of packaging on food quality.

Denmark

The most recent relevant Act is No.174, Section 7 (April 1950) which provides that vessels, utensils, machines and packaging materials ... or other packaging coming into contact with foodstuffs destined for sale shall be made of such material and be of such nature as not to contaminate or damage the foodstuff. Specifically, packaging is covered by the National Health Service, which issued in July 1962 a "Circular on the Use of Plastics in Contact with Food and Drinking Water". This gives details of the requirements for cheese, pre-packed or cut meat products, milk and potable water and specifications for the plastics themselves. A short positive list of additives was also included. Control of the Act is by the National Health Service who obtain technical advice from the National Food Institute and the Toxiological Laboratory in Copenhagen.

In Denmark, plastics for sale, should if possible conform to the requirements of
the 1962 circular. If this is not possible or convenient, conformity with other
major foreign legislation or codes of practice (e.g. United Kingdom or United
States of America) is usually accepted.

Spain

The current law on food contact materials, covers, toys, school equipment, coatings,
utensils and all food contact uses including food itself is the Spanish Food Code
promulgated in Decree 2484 (1967). Specific requirements for plastics are in
Section 2.04.02 which in Sub-Section 3(a) states " ... plasticised papers, which
observe the conditions established in part (a) ... the plastics used shall be
limited by the nature of their residues ... ". Sub-Section 5 states that
"Macromolecular components , such as rubber and its derivatives, plastics materials
and varnishes, which comply with the tests and applicational tests relevant to their
end-use may be made of the following materials:

(a) Natural or synthetic resins or high polymers resistant to degradation during
    conversion or use,

(b) Soluble volatiles, which leave no residue in the finished product,

(c) Non-toxic plasticising monomers or high polymers,

(d) Authorised stabilisers, drying agents, pigments and colourants,

(e) Non-toxic improvers and fillers,

(f) Permitted antioxidants.

In Section 2.04.03 the use of the following substances are forbidden: zinc,
cadmium compounds in food wrappings and non-virgin textiles for food wrapping uses.
Also forbidden are "plastics materials that can change the organoleptic properties
of foodstuffs or yield toxic substances".

No positive lists have been issued in Spain. Law enforcement is by local public
health authorities and police.

In general, plastics merchants wishing to comply with Spanish legislation should
ensure avoidance of zinc and cadmium compounds, also systems liable to produce
organoleptic problems. The use of regrind or reused polymer should also be
avoided. Conformity with a widely accepted foreign legislation such as United
Kingdom or United States of America is strongly recommended.

The situation in various other countries is reviewed below:

Country	Relevant Law	Items Covered
Austria	a) Food Law (1951) modified 19/10/66 (published by Federal Health Journal No.235). b) Food Utensils Decree 1960 (Federal Health Journal No.258) c) Decree under General Food Law covering colourants in food utensils and packaging paper.	Articles contacting food-stuffs (tableware, food utensils, cooking equipment, packaging etc)
East Europe (including Bulgaria, Czechoslovakia, German Democratic Republic, Poland, Rumania and Yugoslavia.	State Controlled.	
Canada	Food and Drugs Act RS1927 C76 and subsequent amendments up to June 1969. See regulation B23 29/5/68 division 23 Food Packaging Materials.	Food and Substances mixed with food. Packages.

Key Quotations	Positive Lists	Seeking Approval
"Plastics or rubbers are prohibited if the food contacting them is changed in such a way that it becomes a hazard to health."	Limited list for plastics and additives.	Approval likely to be given if prior approval can be shown by Food and Drug Administration (USA), UK Code of Practics or Federal German Bundesgesundheitamt (BGH).
		Individual merchants can obtain information on State's requirements by direct communication. Regarding imported goods, the State often requires conformity with the FDA or West German Bundesgesundheitamt (BGA) Regulations. Poland is an exception, details of requirements obtainable from the State Import Organisation, Poliglob S.A.
"No person shall sell an article of food that a) has in or upon it any poisonous or harmful substance. b) is adulterated or c) was packaged under insanitary conditions". "No person shall sell any food in a package that may yield to its contents any substance that may be injurous to the health of a consumer of the food."	Positive list for PVC.	Policing of food safety by inspectors organised under the Federal Food and Drugs Directorate (FDD) who can authorise the use of plastics in contact with food either on the basis of written approval or on the basis of Common Law or the equivalent sections B23 and B23001 of the Food and Drugs Act. In Canada, a merchant should either obtain FDD approval or show that the package is safe according to Common Law and conform to the FDA regulations (USA).

Country	Relevant Law	Items Covered
Australia	In State of Victoria Health Act 1958 and amendments (similar to UK Food and Drug Act 1955) Food and Drugs Standard Regulations 1966 of the Department of Health, Victoria.	Food, Toys (packaging not specifically mentioned)
New Zealand	Food and Drugs Act 1969. Plastics in contact with food Regulation No.42 (b) under Section 20.	Packaging and food contact materials.
South Africa	Food, Drugs and Disinfectant Act No.54, 1972.	Plastics in contact with food.
India	Prevention of Food Adulteration Act (No.37) 1954 with amendments up to 1968.	Utensils, packaging materials plastics (Section 2, 1954 Act).

Key Quotations	Positive Lists	Seeking Approval
"No package or container or appliance shall be used which may yield to its food contents any poisonous or injurous substance."	positive list.	Merchant should meet requirements on toxic metals, butylated hydroxy toluene and ensure that packaging meets requirements of FDA (USA), UK Code of Practice or Federal German Bundes-gesundheitamt.
Migration limits quoted for tin, arsenic, lead, copper, zinc, and selenium.	Negative Lists issued.	A merchant should ensure by product would meet the UK Code of Practice and the New Zealand Food and Drugs Act limits for migration of metallic residues from the plastic into the food.
Government Notice R.1238 5/8/70 (Regulation under 1929 Food, Drugs and Disinfectant Act) "No package, wrapper, container or appliance used in connection with food shall be of such a composition or nature as to yield to its food contents or to food with which it comes into contact, any unwholesome, injurous or poisonous substances."		No detailed regulations issued covering plastics in contact with food. To ensure conformity with the legislation a merchant should take reasonable precautions to avoid any toxic hazards that may be introduced through plastics in contact with food. In many cases compliance with the USA Food and Drugs Administration regulations would be regarded as satisfactory by the authorities.
Requirements on sanitation, presence of poisonous on deleterious substances, colouring matter prohibited preservatives and permitted preser- vatives in excess of prescribed limits.		No detailed specifications issued on quality require- ments of plastic packaging required to meet the Act. It is recommended that plastics for use in contact with food in India should conform to at least one of the well known national specifications such as those of USA, UK, France or West Germany.

Country	Relevant Law	Items Covered
Japan	Food Sanitary Law No.233, 1947 and Laws 113 and 213, 1953 updated 1969.	Article 9 on Food Sanitary Law packaging and food contact.
Latin America, Argentine, Brazil, Chile, Cost Rica, Dominican Republi c, El Salvador, Guatamala, Nicaragua, Panama, Paraguay, Peru, Trinidad and Venezuela.	Latin American Food Code 1965, Second edition.	Contact with food utensils, receptacles, containers, wrappers and machinery.

Key Quotations	Positive Lists	Seeking Approval
"Apparatus on containers or packages apt to injure human health being in contact with food and additives and thus causing injurous influence thereto, shall neither be sold, manufactured ... or imported for sale."		Law gives no specific guidance to quality of plastic required a merchant should seek approval from the appropriate city or provincial health labora-tory, quoting all foreign approvals. If these include USA Food and Drugs Admin-istration, Japanese approval is almost certain.
Section dealing specifically with plastics (Article 58) states, "all utensils ... , that come into contact with food must ... not yield harmful substances or substances capable or contaminating or modifying any organo-leptic characteristics of the food".		Approval usually given by Ministry of Health. No specific regulations yet issued regarding plastics for contact with food. Merchant should supply, analytical migration, tainting trials data and information of foreign approvals, especially USA Food and Drug Administration and West German Bundesges-heitamt.

REFERENCES

1. *Second Report of the Toxicity Sub-committee of the Main Technical Committee of The British Plastics Federation,* with Methods of Analysis of Representative Extractants, The British Plastics Federation ,47-48 Piccadilly, London, W.1. 1962.

2. *United States Federal Register Title 21 Food and Drugs.* Chapter 1. Food and Drug Administration Department of Health and Education and Welfare. Part 121. Food Additives: Subpart F, Food Additives resulting from contact with containers or equipment and food additives otherwise affecting food; Sections 121, 2501 (polypropylene) and 121, 2510 (polyethylene). Amendments published in the Federal Register. Pages 13.3, 13.4 and 13.8 – March 13th, 1963. 28 F.R. 2445 and Pages 13.5, 13.6 and 13.7 – February 10th, 1962. 27 F.R. 1252. 121.51 Pages 4.1 to 4.6 November 28th, 1964. 29 F.R. 15916 (Subpart A. Food Additives), 121, 2526 Pages 28 to 28.1 February 25th 1965, 30 F.R. 2431 (Subpart F. Food Additives), 121, 2526 Page 28.2. February 18th, 1966. 31 F.R. 2897 (Subpart F. Food Additives). 121. 2526 Page 28.3. July 2nd, 1966. 31. F.R.9106 (Subpart F. Food Additives) 121.2526 Page 28.3a February 8th, 1966. 31 F.R. 2476 (Subpart F. Food Additives) 121.2526 Page 28.4 January 28th, 1966. (Subpart F. Food Additives). 121.2526 Page 28.5 January 28th, 1966. 31.F.R.1149 (Subpart F. (Subpart F. Food Additives) 121.2526 Page 28.6 January 18th, 1966. 31.F.R. 560 (Subpart F. Food Additives) 121.2526 Page 28.7 February 25th, 1965. 30.F.R. 2431 (Subpart F. Food Additives)

3. Food and Drug Administration (1967), *Code of Federal Regulations,* Chapter 1, Part 121, Sections 121, 2514 and 121, 2526 pp 239 and 269. U.S. Government Printing Office, Washington D.C.

4. Garlanda, T. and Masaero, H., *La Chimica e l'Industria,* 78 No.9 (1966).

5. Masaero, M and Garlanda, T., *La Chimica e l'Industria,* No.47, 973 (1965).

6. Robinson, L. and Becker, K., *Kunststoffe* 55, 233 (1965).

7. Robinson, L. and Becker, K., *Kunstoffe* 55, 233 (1965).

8. Morton, R.A. and Stubbs, A.L., *Analyst* 71, 348 (1946).

9. Drushel, H.V. and Sommers, A.L., *Anal. Chem.* 36, 836 (1964).

10. Uhde, W.J., Waggon, H., Zydek, G. and Koehler, U. *Deutsch Lebensmittelhdsch,* 65, 271 (1969).

11. Wildbrett, G., Evers, K.W. and Kiermeier, F., *Z.Lebensmittelunters. U-Forsch.* 137, 365 (1968).

220   References

12.   Wildbrett, G., Evers, K.W. and Kiermeier, F., *Z.Lebensmittelunters. U-Forsch.*
      142, 205 (1970).

13.   Wildbrett, G., Evers, K.W. and Kiermeier, F., *Fetter Seifen Anstrmittel,*
      71, 330 (1969).

14.   Daues, G.W. and Hamner, W.F., *Anal. Chem.*29, 1035 (1957).

15.   Bird, W.L. and Hale, C.H.,*Anal. Chem.* 24, 58 (1952).

16.   Shapras, P. and Claver, G.C., *Anal. Chem.* 36, 2282 (1964).

17.   Adcock, L.H. and Hope, W.G. *Analyst* 95, 968 (1970).

18.   Newman, E.J. and Jones, P.D. *Analyst* 94, 406 (1966).

19.   Suk, V. and Malat, M. *Chemist Analyst* 45, 30 (1956).

20.   Ross W.J. and White, J.C. *Analyst Chem.* 33, 421 (1961).

21.   Koch, J. and Figge, K. *Z. Lebensmittelunters-u-Forsch* 147, 8 (1971).

22.   Wieczorek, H. *Deutsch Dt. Lebensmittrdsch.* 66, 92 (1970).

23.   Wieczorek, H. *Analytical Abstracts* 19, 348 (1970).

24.   Slezewska, L. *Roczn. panst. Zakl. Hig.* 23, 417 (1972).

25.   Colson, A.F. *Analyst* 88, 26 (1963).

26.   Colson. A.F. *Analyst* 88, 791 (1963).

27.   Colson, A.F. *Analyst* 90, 35 (1965).

28.   Salvage, T. and Dixon, J.F. *Analyst* 90, 24 (1965).

29.   Mann, L.T. *Anal. Chem.* 35, 2179 (1963).

30.   Johnson, C.A. and Leonard, M.A. *Analyst* 86, 101 (1961).

31.   Yoshizaki, T. *Anal. Chem.* 35, 2177 (1963).

32.   Waggon, H. and Uhde, W.D. *Ernährungsforschung* 16, 227 (1971).

33.   Italian Ministry of Health. Health regulations for packages, wrappings,
      containers and utensils intended for contact with foodstuffs or with
      substances for personal use. In Italian. *Gazetta Ufficiale,*
      7 March, No. 64 p. 18 (1963).

34.   Franck, R., *Kunstostoffe im Lebensmittelverkehr. Empfehlungen der
      Kunststoff-Kommission des Bundesgesundheitsamtes. Teil B.* 7th issue, p.6,
      Carl Heymanns Verlag KG, Köln (1967).

35.   Netherlands Ministry of Social Affairs and Public Health. Draft packaging
      and food utensils regulation (Food Law), (3rd version). In Dutch.
      Staatsblad van het Konindrijk der Nederlanden, 25 July, No. 143. (1968).

36. Figge, K. *Food Cosmet. Toxicol*, 10, 815 (1972).

37. Figge, K. *Migration von Hilfsstoffen der Kunststoffnerarbeitung aus Folien, in Nahrungsfette und Fettsimulantein*. Paper read at the meeting, "Aus den Arbeit von Chemischen Forschungslaborotorien" of Ortverland Hamburg GDCL" on 1st February in Hamburg, (1972).

38. Figge, K. *Angew. Chem*. 83, 901 (1971).

39. Figge, K. *Kunststoffe* 61, 832 (1971).

40. Figge, K. Eder, S.R. and Piater, H. *Dt. LebensmittRdsch*. 68, 359 (1972).

41. Figge, K. and Piater, H. *Dt. LebensmittRdsch* 67, 9 (1971 a).

42. Figge, K. and Piater, H. *Dt. LebensmittRdsch* 67, 47 (1971 b).

43. Figge, K. and Piater, H. *Dt. LebensmittRdsch* 67, 110 (1971 c).

44. Figge, K. and Piater, H. *Dt. LebensmittRdsch* 67, 154 (1971 d).

45. Figge, K. and Piater, H. *Dt. LebensmittRdsch* 67, 235 (1971 e).

46. Figge, K. and Piater, H. *Dt. LebensmittRdsch* 68, 313 (1972).

47. Figge, K. and Schoene, J. *Dt. LebensmittRdsch* 66, 281 (1970).

48. Piater, H. and Figge. K. Migration von Hilfsstoffen der Kunststoffverarbeitung aus Folien in Flussige und feste Fette bzw. Simulantien. VIII. Mitteilung: Vergleich der gravimetrisch bestimmten Rückstände der Extraktionslosungen mit den tatsächlich extrahierten Additivmengen. (1971).

49. vom Bruck, C.G., Figge, K., Piater, H. and Wolf, V. *Dt. LebensmittRdsch* 67, 444 (1971).

50. vom Bruck, C.G., Figge, K. and Wolf, V. *Dt. LebensmittRdsch* 66, 253 (1970).

51. Figge, K. *Food Cosmet. Toxicol*. 10, 815 (1972).

52. Figge, K. *Synthese eines radiokohlenstoff-markierten Organozinn-Stabilisators zur Bestimmung von Migrationsvorgängen*. Paper read at the meeting, "Präparative Radiochemie" of "Gesellschaft Deutscher Chemiker" (GDCh) on 5-6 September in Lindau/Bodensee (1968).

53. Figge, K. *J.Labell Compounds* 5, 122 (1969).

54. Ministre de la Santé Publique. Circulaire du 12 Septembre 1963 relative aux demandes d'autorisation d'emploi de substances chimiques destinées à être introduites dans les aliments ou utilisées dans les matériaux mis aux contact des aliments. *Journal officiel*, 26 September (1963).

55. Emptehlungen der Kunststoff-Kommission des Bundesgusundheitsamtes (B.G.A.) I. Mitteilung, *Bundesgesundheitsblatt* 4, 189 and 10, (1967).

56. Van der Heide, R.F. *Packaging* 54 (1966).

57. Van der Heide, R.F., *The Safety for Health of Plastics Food Packaging Materials* (Utrecht 1964) page 32.

58. Pfab, W., *Z Lebensmittel-Unter-u-Forsch*. 115, 428 (1961).

59. Strodtz, N.H. and Henry, R.E., *"Industrial Methods of the Analysis of Food Additives"*. New York (1961) Page 85

60. Phillips, J. and Marks G.C., *Brit. Plastics*, 34, 319 and 385, (1961).

61. American Society for Testing Materials (ASTM) Method No. F.34-63 T. Pfab, W., *Dt. Lebensmitt Rdsch*.64, 281 (1968) and J. Assoc of agric-Chemists 47, 177 (1964), also *Fluckiger E and Henscher, H., Dtsch Molkerei - Ztg* 99, 848 (1969).

62. Koch, J. and Figge, K., *Dt. Lebensmitt-Rdsch*, 71, 170 (1975)

63. Figge, K. and Koch, J., *Food Cosmet Toxicol*, 11, 975 (1973).

64. Van der Heide *"The Safety for Health of Plastics Food Packaging Materials Principles and Chemical Methods"*, Kemink En Zoon N V - Utrecht (1964).

65. Waggon, H., Jehle, D. and Uhde, W.J., *Nahrung*, 13, 343   (1969)

66. Waggon, H., Uhde, W.J. and Zydek, G., *Z. Lebensmittel unters u-Forsch* 138, 169 (1968)

67. Figge, K and Zeman, A., *Kunststoffe* 63, 543 (1973)

68. Phillips, I. and Marks, G.C., *British Plastics*, 34, 319 (1961)

69. Phillips, I. and Marks, G.C. *British Plastics*, 34, 385 (1961)

70. Koch, J., *Dt. LebensmittRdsch* 68, 401 (1972)

71. Koch, J., *Dt. LebensmittRdsch* 68, 404 (1972)

73. Uhde, W.J., Waggon, H and Koehler, U., *Nahrung* 12, 813 (1968)

74. Uhde, W.J., Waggon, H. and Koehler, U., *Analytical Abstracts* 18, 327 (1970) *Plaste Kautsch* 15, 630 (1968)

75. Uhde, W.J. and Waggon, H. *Dt. Lebensmittell-Rdsch* 67, 257 (1971)

76. Uhde, W.J. and Waggon, H., *Nahmung* 12, 825 (1968)

77. Uhde, W.J. and Waggon, H., *Analytical Abstracts*, 18, 2024 (1970)

78. Sampaolo, A., Rossi, L., Binetti, R., Cesolari, C. and Fava, G., *Raoss. Chimo* 24, 3 (1972)

79. Hilton, C.L., *Analytical Abstracts* 7, 4893 (1960)

80. Wadelin, O., *Analytical Abstracts* 4, 982 (1957)

81. Piacentini, R., *Industria Gomma* 16, 46 (1972)

82. Bergner, K.G. and Berg, H., *Dt. LebensmittRdsch* 68, 282 (1972)

83. Rohleder, K. and von Bruch-hauser, B., *Dt. LebensmittRdsch* 68, 180 (1972)

84. Koch, J., *Dt. LebenmittRdsch* 70, 209 (1974)

85. Figge, K., *Kunststoffe* 61, 832 (1971)

86. Figge, K. and Zeman, A., *Kunststoffe* 63, 543 (1973)

87. Figge, K. and Koch, J., private communication

88. Figge, K. and Bieber, W.D., private communication

89. Figge, K., *Verpackungs-Rundschau* 8, 59 (1975)

90. Figge, K., *Food Cosmet Toxicology* 11, 963 (1973)

91. Figge, K., *Bundesgesundhbl* 24, 27 (1975)

92. Figge, K., *Dt. LebensmittRdsch* 71, 129 (1975)

93. Figge, K and Koch, J., *Fette Seifen Anstrichmittel* 77, 184 (1975)

94. Aldershoff, W.G., *Annali Ist sup. Sanita* 8, 550 (1972)

95. Baumgartner, E., *Kunststoffe-Plastics* 15, 3 (1968)

96. Federal Health Office, Berne *Schweizerisches Lebensmittelbuch, Vorentwurf, V. Auflage, Band II, Kap, 48-Kunststoffe* (1966)

    Figge ,K. Paper read at the meeting "Praparative Radiochemie" of "Gesellschaft Deutscher Chemiker" (GDCh) on 5-6 September in Lindau/Bodensee (1968).

97. Italian Ministry of Health, Ministerial Decree of 15 April 1966. *Gazzetta Ufficiale* 7 May, no. 111, p. 2295 (1961)

98. United States Code of Federal Regulations. Section 121, 2501

99. United States Code of Federal Regulations. Section 121, 2514

100. Figge, K. and Piater, H., *Dt. LebensmittRdsch* 68, 313 (1972)

101. BITMP (Bureaux Internationaux Techniques des Matières Plastiques) *Dt. LebensmittRdsch* 68, 37 (1972)

102. Brugger, R., Doctorial dissertation University of Bern (1971)

103. de Wilde, J.H. *Dt. LebesmittRdsch* 61, 369 (1966)

104. Fluckiger, E. and Rentsch, C., *Alimenta* 7, 41 (1968)

105. Robinson-Görnhardt, L., *Kunststoffe* 47, 265 (1957)

106. Robinson-Görnhardt, L., *Kunststoffe* 48, 463 (1958)

107. Unpublished work

108. BITMP (Bureaux Internationaux Techniques des Matières Plastiques). *Determination de la migration des constituants des materiaux destinés a être mis au contact des denrées alimentaires ayant un contact gras.* Report Brüssel. (1971)

109. Pfab, W., *Annali lst. sup. Sanità* 8, 385 (1972)

110. van Battum, D. and Rijk, M.A.H., *Annali lst. sup. Sanità* 8, 421 (1972)

111. Wildrett, G., Evers, K.W. and Kiermeier, F. *Z. Lebenmittel unters. u-Forsch* 142, 205 (1970)

112. Koch, J., *Dt. LebensmittRdsch*. 68, 216, 401 and 404. (1972)

113. Figge, K., *Fd. Cosmet. Toxicol.* 10, 815 (1972)

114. Figge, K., Eder, S.R. and Piater, H., *Dt. LebensmittRdsch*, 68, 359 (1972)

115. Figge, K., *Kunststoffe* 61, 832 (1971)

116. Figge, K. and Piater, H., *Dt. LebensmittRdsch* 67, 47, 110, 154 and 235 (1971)

117. Piater, H. and Figge, K., *Dt. LebensmittRdsch* 67, 265 (1971)

118. vom Bruck, C.G., Figge, K., Piater, H. and Wolf, V., *Dt. LebensmittRdsch* 67, 444 (1971)

119. Figge, K., *Dt. LebensmittRdsch* 7, 253 (1973)

120. Koch, J. and Kröne, R., *Dt. LebensmittRdsch* 8, 291 (1975)

121. Pfab, W., *Dt. LebensmittRdsch* 68, 350 (1972)

122. von Battum, D. and Rijk, M.A.H., *Annali lst. sup. Sanità* 8, 421 (1972)

123. Phillips, A.M., *J. Am. Oil Chem. Soc.* 50, 21 (1973)

124. Hartman, K.T. and Rose, L.C., *J. Am. Oil Chem. Soc.* 47, 7 (1970)

125. Lemieszek-Chadorowska, K. and Snycerski, A., *Roczn Panst. Zakl, Hy.* 20, 261 (1969)

126. Valdehita de Vincente, Maria and Teresa, Vicente., *An. Bromat.*, 23, 107 (1971)

127. Schwein, O. and Conroy, O.J, *Ass. Off. Agric. Chem.* 48, 489 (1965)

128. Chiang, Hung-Cheh., Tseng, Ren-Gun., *J. Pharm. Sci.* 58, 1552 (1969)

129. Lehman, G. and Moran, M., *Z. Lebensmittel unters. u-Forsch* 145, 344 (1971)

130. Vigneron, P.Y. and Spicht, P., *Revue fr. Cps. Gras.* 17, 295 (1970)

131. Pino, A.M.I., Leiro, J.V. and Schmidt-Hebbel, H., *Grasas Aceit* 20, 129 (1969)

132. McBride, H.D. and Evans, D.H., *Anal. Chem.* 45, 446 (1973)

133. Köhler, U., Waggon, H. and Uhde, W.J., *Plaste. Kautsch.* 15, 630 (1968)

134. Takahashi, D.M. *J. Ass. Off. Analyt. Chem.* 53, 39 (1970)

135. Takahashi, D.M., *Anal. Abstracts* 17. 3063 (1969)

136. Takemura, I. *Japan Analyst* 20, 61 (1971)

137. Halot, D., *Chim. Analyt.* 53, 776 (1971)

138. Lee, S.C., *Chemistry Taipei* 43, 155 (1968)

139. Lee, S.C., *Analytical Abstracts* 14, 7864 (1967)

140. Roos, J.B., *Fette Seifen Anstrichmittel* 60, 1160 (1958)

141. Biefer, K.W. and Hadorn, H., *Mitt Gebiete Lebensmittelunters. Hyg. (Berne)* 47, 445 (1956)

142. Gander, F., *Fette Seifen. Anstrichmittel* 57, 423 (1955)

143. Gander, F., *Fette Seifen. Anstrichmittel* 58, 506 (1956)

144. Brown, F. and Baxter, K.L., *Chem. and Ind.* 633 (1951)

145. Brown, F. and Baxter, K.L., *Biochem. J.* 51, 237 (1952)

146. ter Heide, R., *Fette Seifen Anstrichmittel* 60, 360 (1958)

147. Zipp, J.W.H., *Rec. Trav. Chim. Pays-Bas* 75, 1053, 1060, 1089, 1129, 1155 (1956)

148. Stahl, E., *Chem. Zeitung* 82, 323 (1958)

149. Seher, A., *Fette Seifen Anstrichmittel* 61, 345 (1959)

150. Seher, A., *Fette Seifen Anstrichmittel* 60, 1144 (1958)

INDEX

30,974

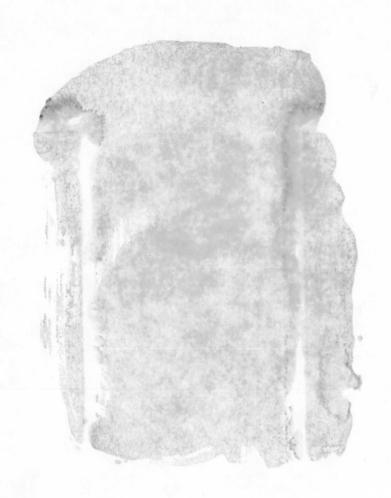